Your Pregnancy and Childbirth

Celia McInnes, BA
Penny Tripp

HARRAP

London

Published 1989 by
Harrap Books Limited
19-23 Ludgate Hill, London EC4M 7PD
By arrangement with Amanuensis Books Ltd

ISBN 0 245-55068-2

This book was designed and produced by
Amanuensis Books Ltd
12 Station Road
Didcot
Oxfordshire OX11 7LL
UK

Cover design: Roger King Graphic Studios
Editorial and art director: Loraine Fergusson
Senior editor: Lynne Gregory
Editor: Laila Grieg-Gran
Illustration: Loraine Fergusson, Ron Freeborn, Lynne Gregory,
David Gifford

Prime Health Ltd, a subsidiary of Municipal General Insurance Ltd (MGI)
has contributed to the cost of this publication.

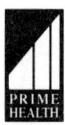

The information contained in this book has been obtained from professional
medical sources and every care has been taken to ensure that it is consistent with
current medical practice. However, it is intended only as a guide to current medical
practice and not as a substitute for the advice of your medical practitioner which
must, on all occasions, be taken.

Contents

Conception

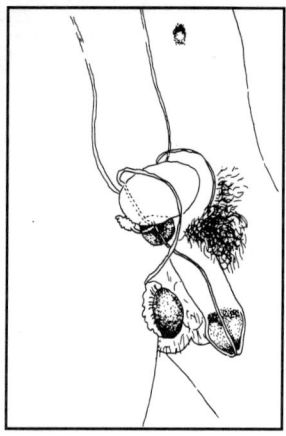

Spermatozoa travel up the sperm duct from the testicles which hang outside the body in the scrotum. During ejaculation they are pumped out of the urethra of the penis, high into the female vagina.

A pregnancy begins when two cells join to form the beginnings of a new life. One of these cells comes from a man, the other from a woman and when they join they form a nucleus which contains the blueprint for all the characteristics that will make this new child a unique individual.

The male reproductive system

The main function of the male reproductive organs is to produce healthy spermatozoa (sperm which carry the male reproductive cell) and deliver them into the female reproductive tract as near to the cervix (the neck of the womb) as possible.

However, the male sex organs are also responsible for manufacturing male sex hormones, particularly testosterone which is responsible for the secondary sexual characteristics in men such as the development of pubic and chest hair, a deep voice and broad shoulders.

The scrotum and testicles

The testes (testicles) are made up of thousands of tubes in which the sperm are manufactured. Each testis is oval, about the size of a walnut, and hangs outside the body inside a muscular pouch called the scrotum. The scrotum maintains the testes at a temperature a couple of degrees below body temperature which is essential for the production of sperm. If the surrounding air temperature rises the muscles in the scrotum relax allowing the testes to move further away from the body, and if the surrounding temperature is too cold, the muscles contract and the testes rise closer to the warmth of the body.

If this mechanism is disrupted, for example, by wearing overtight clothing or by sedentary jobs such as long-distance truck driving, there is evidence that a man's fertility can be reduced or even cease altogether. (Hot baths before intercourse were a recognized contraceptive measure during Roman times.)

The penis

The penis is a dual-purpose organ. The urethra (the tube)

which runs down the centre of the penis transports urine from the bladder as well as carrying ejaculated sperm. However, just before ejaculation the urinary entrance is closed off by muscular contractions which prevents any urine coming into contact with the delicate sperm and possibly damaging them.

The penis is made of tissue which contains many small blood compartments. When sexually stimulated, these fill with blood and the engorged penis becomes rigid enabling it to penetrate the vaginal opening of the female.

Ejaculation
When the man reaches orgasm, the muscles of the genitalia (male sex organs) contract rhythmically pumping about three to five millilitres of sperm and seminal fluid (semen) up the urethra and high into the female vagina. The number of sperm emitted ranges between 20 to 300 million.

The semen
The alkaline, rather gelatinous semen (or seminal fluid) is manufactured by the prostate gland and the two Cowper's glands at the base of the penis. The seminal fluid both nourishes and protects the sperm from the acid secretions of the female vagina. After about 15 to 20 minutes it liquefies.

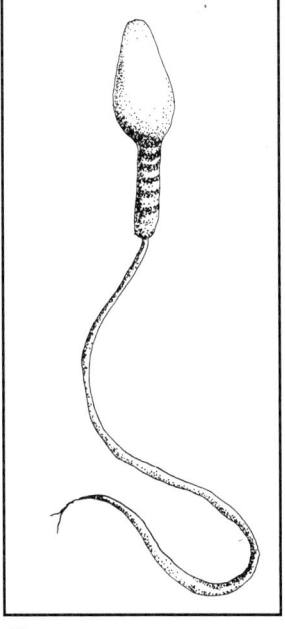

The sperm
Each sperm is about .04 mm long and consists of a head, neck and long, lashing tail. Human sperm are produced continuously by the male in enormous numbers from puberty right through into old age although sperm production does decrease after the age of fifty. This sperm production is called spermatogenesis. Once formed, the sperm gather in a tightly coiled tube called the epididymis to mature before passing, by way of a tube called the vas deferens, to the seminal vesicles where they are stored until ejaculation.

The female reproductive organs
The female body has more to do than just produce an egg. It also has to nurture the resulting embryo and fetus until it is able to support life on its own.

The vagina
The vagina leads from the external female genitalia (the labia majora and labia minora which means the big and little lips) to the cervix (neck of the womb). It is about 10 cm long and made of muscle and elastic tissue, and lined with folds of skin which allow the vagina to stretch as the muscles relax both during sexual excitement to allow the entry of the penis, and later during the birth of a baby. At the entrance to the vagina the folds of skin bunch up to

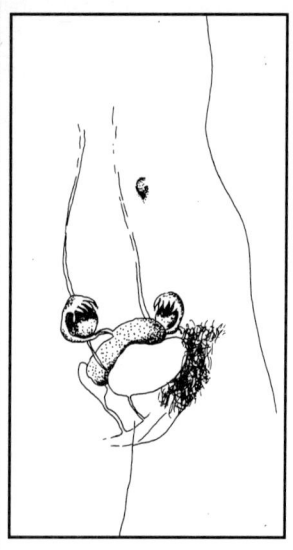

The uterus is a muscular organ which lies behind the bladder and is protected by the pelvic ring.

form the hymen which partly seals off the vagina of a young girl until exercise, handling or intercourse stretches or breaks it. Even then some part may remain until torn further during childbirth after which only a few tags are left behind.

The vagina is normally moist, lubricated by secretions from the cervix and from the Bartholin's glands on each side of the entrance. During sexual stimulation the glands produce extra secretions to further aid the penetration of the penis. Mucus is also produced by glands inside the cervix which alters depending on the stage of the menstrual cycle.

The uterus (womb)

The uterus is pear-shaped and hollow. It is about 10 cm long and 6 cm at its widest point. It is made up of three layers of tissue - an outer membrane, a middle layer of muscle and tissue and an inner layer which is called the endometrium.

The muscles of the middle layer run vertically, horizontally and diagonally and are of the type known as smooth or involuntary muscle. This means that, like the muscles of the bowel, they cannot be consciously controlled. They do actually contract and relax throughout a woman's life but she would not be aware of this except sometimes during menstruation and in late pregnancy and labour. They are among the strongest muscles in the body. After holding a full-term baby they will shrink by two-thirds within minutes of the birth and be back to their original size within six weeks.

The endometrium is the layer which lines the uterus. It is the top layer of this blood-rich tissue that is shed by the uterus during menstruation only to build up again over the next month. If on the other hand fertilization takes place, it is into the endometrium that the embryo implants itself.

The cervix

This is the lower part of the uterus which is made up of a ring of muscle and forms the neck of the womb. Firmer and harder, this forms a passage about 4 cm long down into the vagina. This opening becomes wider as ovulation approaches shutting down as soon as the egg has been released. The cervix contains crypts which produce cervical mucus. Leading up to ovulation the mucus is produced in greater quantities and has an elastic, slippery quality. This mucus is able to nourish the sperm and store them for up to three days in the cervical crypts until ovulation. After ovulation the cervical mucus changes and forms a physical barrier against the sperm. Throughout pregnancy the cervix remains tightly closed and plugged with mucus (when this plug is expelled early on during the first stage of labour it is sometimes referred to as the 'show').

The fallopian tubes

Named after the sixteenth-century Italian anatomist Fallopius, these paired tubes are also called the uterine tubes or oviducts. They are about 10 cm long and run from the upper and outer corners of the uterus towards the ovaries where they open out into funnel shapes fringed with many delicate fronds known as fimbriae.

When an egg is released from one of the ovaries, the fimbriae waft it towards the opening of the fallopian tube. Once in the tube it begins to descend towards the uterus, and it is in the tube itself that fertilization of the ovum by the sperm actually takes place. The ovum is moved down the tube by contractions of muscles within the tube wall as well as by the movements of hair-like cilia.

The mucous membrane which lines the tubes also nourishes both the egg and the sperm while they are in transit which in the case of a fertilized egg will be about seven days. Should the fertilized egg take longer than seven days to pass through to the uterus there is a danger that it will embed itself there rather than in the uterus. This can result in a tubal or ectopic pregnancy which cannot succeed and can lead to serious complications.

The ovaries

The ovaries are two glands about the size and shape of large almonds. They lie within the pelvis near the funnel-shaped end of each tube. The ovaries play a crucial role in

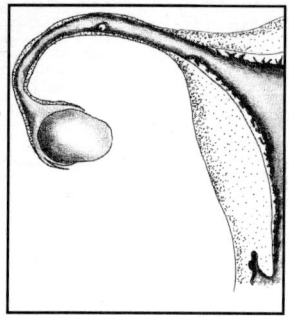

Fertilization occurs not in the uterus, but inside the fallopian tube itself. The fertilized ovum is already dividing and subdividing by the time it reaches the lining of the uterus and implants.

the control of the fertility cycle of a woman as well as producing a viable ovum approximately every 28 days from puberty to the menopause.

A woman is born with all the eggs she will ever have already in her ovaries (between four to five million) but by the time she reaches puberty many of these have been absorbed leaving about half a million eggs in the ovaries. Each month between ten to a hundred immature ova begin to ripen, but at the time of ovulation only one of these will reach maturity and be released. (If two are released simultaneously a woman may conceive unidentical twins; if a single ovum is fertilized and splits, identical twins are conceived.)

The ovaries also manufacture the female sex hormones estrogen and progesterone which control the development of a woman's secondary sexual characteristics - wide hips, breasts and pubic hair - as well as controlling the fertility cycle. Normally the ovaries operate on alternate months, but if one is damaged or missing, the other takes over and produces an egg every month as well as all the required hormones.

Ovulation

Stimulated by the complex pattern of hormonal action in the body, the ripening egg develops within a pea-like follicle on the surface of the ovary. The follicle ruptures releasing the ovum which is wafted towards the nearby fallopian tube.

The empty follicle is known as the corpus luteum ('yellow body' because of its colour). If fertilization occurs the corpus luteum maintains the pregnancy for the next six to ten weeks until the hormones released by the developing placenta take over.

Fertilization

Although ovulation occurs month after month, fertilization can only happen if an egg and sperm come together at just the right time.

The egg is released into the fallopian tube at ovulation,

usually on day 14 of the fertility cycle. An ovum is fertilizable for only about 12 hours after ovulation after which time it is reabsorbed into the body. However, because the sperm can live in the cervical crypts for up to three days, the fertility period of a woman is much longer than 12 hours.

A woman with a regular 28-day cycle is at her most fertile between day 11 and day 15, so in order to maximize her chances of conception, she should plan intercourse during these days.

It has been estimated that it takes the sperm about an hour to travel up from the cervix to the end of the fallopian tube but of the millions deposited, only ten percent will reach the safety of the cervical canal. Of the rest, up to 20% will be damaged or abnormal in some way before ejaculation which makes them unable to swim far or fast enough and they die. In fact, should an abnormal sperm manage to reach an egg, it cannot usually fertilize it.

When the sperm encounters the egg, hundreds cluster around it but only one will enter. As it strikes the surface of the ovum, the head of the sperm opens up releasing a special enzyme which dissolves the gelatinous outer membrane (the zona pellucida), but the moment it enters rapid chemical changes alter the surface of the ovum and prevent any more sperm from entering. The powerful tail that has propelled the sperm this far remains on the outside of the egg as only the head enters and moves towards the nucleus of the ovum. The union of the sperm nucleus and the ovum nucleus is the moment of fertilization. Joined they make a full complement of chromosomes, and this now single cell is the beginning of a new life.

Implantation

The fertilized egg moves down the fallopian tube, its new cell already beginning to divide and sub-divide long before it enters the uterus about three days after fertilization. Within six or seven days of fertilization the egg embeds itself in the lining of the uterus, the endometrium. It is only the size of a pinhead, but finger-like projections grow out into the endometrium to begin the formation of the placenta.

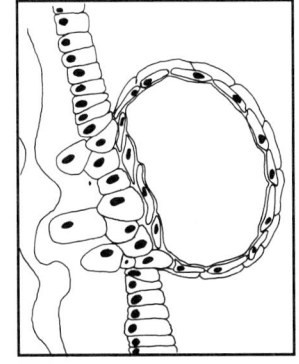

When the fertilized ovum reaches the endometrium, fronds of cells reach out and become embedded in the endometrial lining of the uterus. As these cells further divide and subdivide, so the placenta is formed which will nourish the developing embryo.

The fert

The fertility, or menstrual, cycle is regulated by a series of changes in the pattern of hormone secretions over a period of between 21 and 35 days, the average being a 28-day cycle.

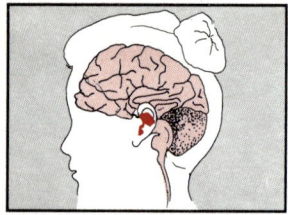

The pituitary gland sits at the base of the brain just between the ears and acts as a controller, stimulating the ovaries to produce estrogen and progesterone, but the pituitary gland itself is affected by hormones from another gland embedded in the base of the brain known as the hypothalamus. As the hypothalamus is so closely connected with other areas of the brain, messages from the brain can affect whether the stimulating hormones are produced at all. This explains why emotional factors can affect ovulation and menstruation - stress, such as anxiety about conceiving, can result in a woman not ovulating at all. Similarly, the fertility cycle can be disrupted by rapid movement through time zones (i.e. accompanying jet lag) and by weight loss as in those suffering from anorexia.

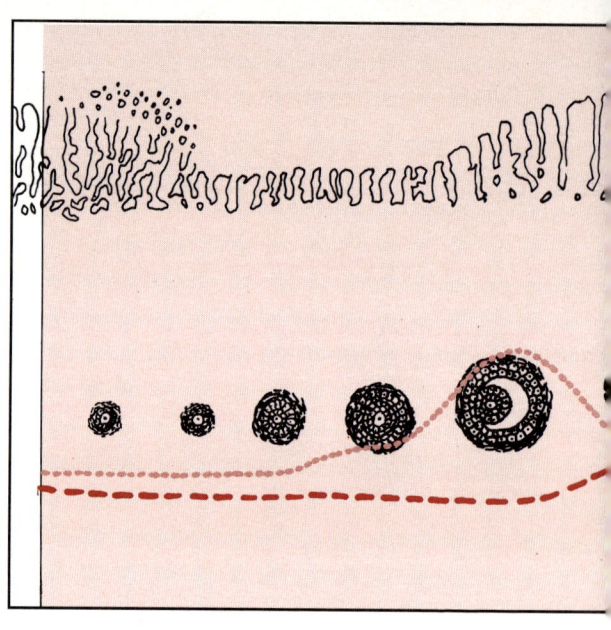

The estrogen phase

The first day of bleeding is regarded as the first day of the menstrual cycle. Bleeding lasts for an average of four to five days and, even in those who have a longer bleeding time, 90% of blood is lost during the first three days. At this stage of the cycle the ovaries are usually relatively inactive, and circulating levels of estrogen and progesterone are low. However, because levels of estrogen and progesterone are low at this stage in the cycle, the pituitary gland releases increasing quantities of follicle stimulating hormone (FSH). FSH causes several follicles to begin ripening in the ovary. Each follicle consists of an immature ovum surrounded by a layer of cells which now begin to produce estrogen. If levels of FSH rise rapidly, the follicles respond to the stimulus and estrogen is produced quickly making the cycle a short one. If FSH levels rise more gradually, or the follicles are more resistant to stimulation, a longer cycle results.

One of the developing

ty cycle

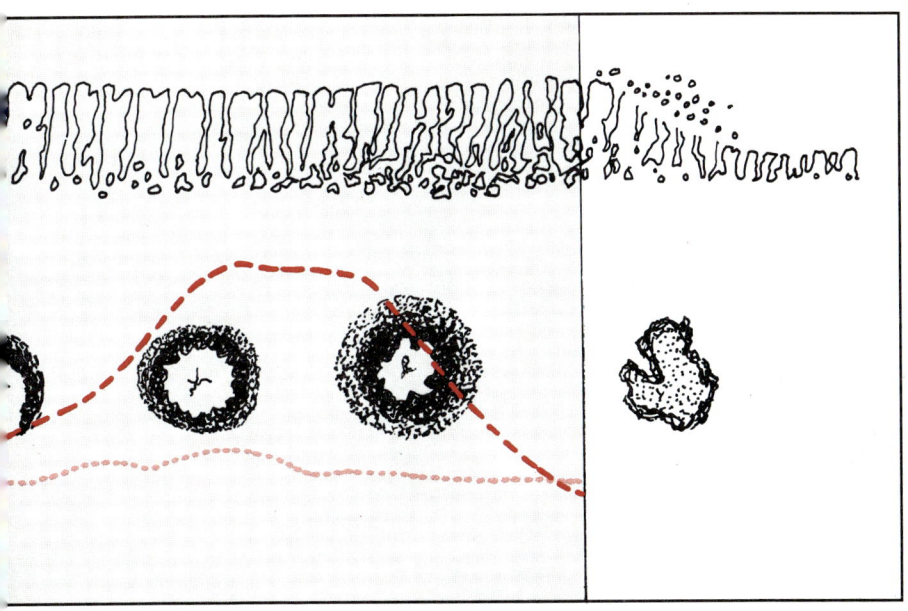

follicles becomes dominant while the others regress. The dominant follicle continues to produce estrogen and the ovum within it develops and grows. The follicle moves towards the surface of the ovary and bursts.

During this stage of the cycle, the endometrial lining of the uterus thickens in preparation to receive the fertilized ovum.

Progesterone phase

The part of the cycle from ovulation to the onset of bleeding is called the progesterone or luteal phase. If fertilization does not occur after ovulation, the corpus luteum produces not just lower levels of estrogen, but also much higher levels of progesterone. This prevents ovulation occurring again during the cycle. If fertilization does not take place, the corpus luteum eventually disintegrates which reduces

the levels of progesterone. As the progesterone levels fall, the endometrial lining of the uterus breaks down and is shed from the body - menstruation begins. The falling hormone levels also allow the hypothalamus to stimulate the pituitary gland to produce follicle stimulating hormone and the cycle begins once again.

Chromosomes and genes

All cells in the human body contain 23 pairs of chromosomes, making 46 in all, except for the sperm and egg which have only 23 chromosomes each. When, upon fertilization, the nuclei of the sperm and egg fuse, their two sets of chromosomes form 46 chromosomes as in all other cells.

Each chromosome consists of thousands of units known as genes made of the chemical DNA (deoxyribonucleic acid) which carry the detailed messages that will determine the whole range of characteristics of the new baby. The genetic structure of the new cell decides from the start what is to be the colour of the hair, pigment of the skin and eyes, height, health and intelligence of the new life. Everything from a happy temperament to a tendency to put on weight is already mapped out with only environmental influences able to make a difference now.

Sex determination

The fusion of the two sets of chromosomes also determines the sex of the baby and it is the sperm that carries the deciding chromosome. All the cells in a woman's body except the eggs carry 44 non-sex chromosomes (which deal with the way the body works and its physical characteristrics) plus two X sex chromosomes. She does not have any Y chromosomes at all. Men, on the other hand, carry an X and a Y chromosome on every cell in their bodies except the sperm of which half will carry an X chromosome, half a Y chromosome.

So, each egg carries 22 non-sex chromosomes plus an X chromosome while a sperm carries 22 non-sex chromosomes plus either an X or a Y chromosome. If the former fuse with the egg the child will have an XX sex chromosome and be female; if the latter the child will have an XY chromosome and be male.

Pregnancy

The very first signs of pregnancy may not always be obvious unless you are familiar with them or are actually on the lookout for them either because you want to be pregnant or because you are anxious that you are.

Amenorrhea (no menstrual period)

Pregnancy is the most common reason for absence of menstruation although not the only one. Certainly for most women a missed period is the first indication that they are pregnant. However, worrying that you may be pregnant is the second commonest cause of amenorrhea.

Partially suppressed periods sometimes occur in early pregnancy and very rarely at monthly intervals throughout a normal pregnancy. They are triggered if a woman's progesterone level is not quite high enough. If you think you are pregnant and your period does not seem to be as heavy as usual, it makes sense to do a home pregnancy test just in case.

Nausea

This is another common symptom of early pregnancy and may come on even before you miss a period. About 50% of pregnant women suffer from nausea which may range from mild symptoms in the morning or the evening when a woman is tired, to severe sickness and vomiting at any time during the day or night. Unpleasant as they are, nausea and vomiting in early pregnancy have no detrimental effects on the developing baby and for most women the symptoms ease off as they enter the fourth month as the body adjusts to the higher hormone levels. However, in some rare cases it can continue right through the pregnancy.

Taste, smell and cravings

Another early indication may be that things taste or smell differently or that you go off certain smells and tastes sometimes to the extent that you cannot bear them. Often this distaste is for ordinary, everyday things like tea, coffee, tobacco and alcoholic drinks. Again, this dislike may lessen as the pregnancy continues, but in the case of alcohol and tobacco, it is a useful way to cut them out altogether. Other women notice a strange metallic taste in their mouths which may manifest itself before a missed period.

You may experience cravings for particular types of food, often surprisingly spicy food such as pickles. As long as eating such food does not upset you, indulge yourself in it in moderation.

Breast changes

Women often feel a tenderness and fullness in their breasts just before a period is due anyway. If the period does not begin and these symptoms persist and become more obvious, then pregnancy is the likely reason. Breast sensations can include great sensitivity around the nipple and tingling through the breasts as well as the normal enlargement as the pregnancy progresses. The breasts enlarge more quickly and noticeably in small-breasted women.

Urination

During pregnancy the urge to urinate happens more frequently. However, it is particularly noticeable during the first few months when a woman may find that she is having to get up two or three times during the night. This settles down during the middle three months but may recur towards the end when increased weight in the abdomen presses on the bladder.

Fatigue and mood swings

Some women suffer from severe and recurring fatigue which overwhelms them without good reason. Others experience an unusual degree of over-emotionalism with sudden irrational changes of mood. Again, changing hormone levels are at fault, but they will settle down.

Tests for pregnancy

To confirm your suspicions you will probably want to carry out a pregnancy test. These work by detecting the presence or absence in your body of the hormone human chorionic gonadotrophin (HCG). This hormone is produced by the body once a fertilized egg has become implanted. It is present in both the blood and the urine.

Blood tests

Immunoassay tests are a fairly new development and can detect even very slight traces of HCG in the blood. This means that accurate results can be obtained earlier. They do, however, require sophisticated equipment and are largely confined to cases where it is important to ascertain pregnancy early. Pregnancy tests are not always accurate (although you are more likely to get a false negative than a false positive result) especially when one has been sought too early, so don't let yourself be carried away with joy or anxiety when you get the first result. Even blood tests have been known to be wrong. The best advice is to wait as long as possible before having the test and at least for a clear two weeks after missing your period. This improves the likelihood of a correct result. However, if you have a negative result but feel you must be pregnant, get the test done again.

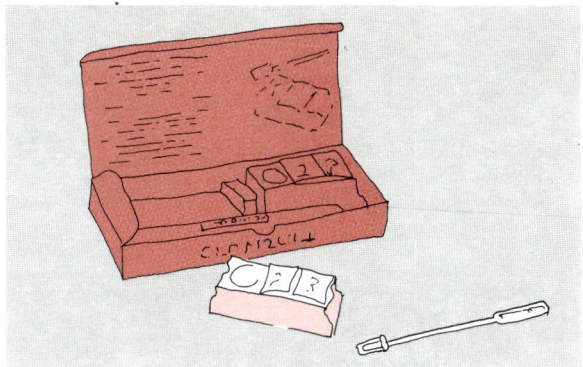

Urine testing

These can usually detect HCG two weeks after your menstrual period was due although some of the home testing kits claim to give a result even earlier. Before this time there is not sufficient HCG to react with the chemicals. Even at two weeks you are advised to use a urine sample taken first thing in the morning when there is the greatest concentration of HCG.

This test can be done by your doctor or at the health centre or family planning clinic where the service is free. Alternatively a chemist can carry out the test, or you can use a home testing kit (illustrated above). These come with careful instructions for use and involve mixing the chemicals supplied with your early morning urine specimen and noting the colour and ring shape which forms in the test tube if the result is positive.

Pelvic examination

A pelvic (internal) examination can confirm a pregnancy about six weeks after the first day of the last period because the uterus enlarges and becomes softer.

Ultrasound

This technique produces echoes which can be added together to produce an image of the fetus on a screen. It can be used to detect pregnancy but is usually reserved for women who need to know urgently that they are pregnant (for example, if there has been a history of miscarriages) because the long-term effects of using ultrasound on the fetus during the early weeks are not yet fully understood although it appears to be quite safe.

When is the baby due?

	1	2	3	4	5	6	7	8	9	10	11	12	13	14
JAN **OCT**	1 / 8	2 / 9	3 / 10	4 / 11	5 / 12	6 / 13	7 / 14	8 / 15	9 / 16	10 / 17	11 / 18	12 / 19	13 / 20	14 / 21
FEB **NOV**	1 / 8	2 / 9	3 / 10	4 / 11	5 / 12	6 / 13	7 / 14	8 / 15	9 / 16	10 / 17	11 / 18	12 / 19	13 / 20	14 / 21
MAR **DEC**	1 / 6	2 / 7	3 / 8	4 / 9	5 / 10	6 / 11	7 / 12	8 / 13	9 / 14	10 / 15	11 / 16	12 / 17	13 / 18	14 / 19
APR **JAN**	1 / 6	2 / 7	3 / 8	4 / 9	5 / 10	6 / 11	7 / 12	8 / 13	9 / 14	10 / 15	11 / 16	12 / 17	13 / 18	14 / 19
MAY **FEB**	1 / 5	2 / 6	3 / 7	4 / 8	5 / 9	6 / 10	7 / 11	8 / 12	9 / 13	10 / 14	11 / 15	12 / 16	13 / 17	14 / 18
JUN **MAR**	1 / 8	2 / 9	3 / 10	4 / 11	5 / 12	6 / 13	7 / 14	8 / 15	9 / 16	10 / 17	11 / 18	12 / 19	13 / 20	14 / 21
JUL **APR**	1 / 7	2 / 8	3 / 9	4 / 10	5 / 11	6 / 12	7 / 13	8 / 14	9 / 15	10 / 16	11 / 17	12 / 18	13 / 19	14 / 20
AUG **MAY**	1 / 8	2 / 9	3 / 10	4 / 11	5 / 12	6 / 13	7 / 14	8 / 15	9 / 16	10 / 17	11 / 18	12 / 19	13 / 20	14 / 21
SEP **JUN**	1 / 8	2 / 9	3 / 10	4 / 11	5 / 12	6 / 13	7 / 14	8 / 15	9 / 16	10 / 17	11 / 18	12 / 19	13 / 20	14 / 21
OCT **JUL**	1 / 8	2 / 9	3 / 10	4 / 11	5 / 12	6 / 13	7 / 14	8 / 15	9 / 16	10 / 17	11 / 18	12 / 19	13 / 20	14 / 21
NOV **AUG**	1 / 8	2 / 9	3 / 10	4 / 11	5 / 12	6 / 13	7 / 14	8 / 15	9 / 16	10 / 17	11 / 18	12 / 19	13 / 20	14 / 21
DEC **SEP**	1 / 7	2 / 8	3 / 9	4 / 10	5 / 11	6 / 12	7 / 13	8 / 14	9 / 15	10 / 16	11 / 17	12 / 18	13 / 19	14 / 20

Once a woman is pregnant, the first thing a couple want to know is when the baby is due. We usually speak of a pregnancy as lasting nine months but in fact the average pregnancy lasts for nine calendar months and seven days, or to be more exact, 280 days from the first day of the last normal menstrual period. It can also be counted out as ten lunar months or 40 weeks and because of the confusion that can arise if 'months' are used when discussing the progression of a pregnancy, most doctors and midwives will stick to using 'weeks'; this also means you can be more precise.

To work out when your baby is due, count back three months and forward a week from the date of the first day of your last period. If this was 6 June, then your estimated date of delivery (EDD) will be 13 March the following year. However, this particular calculation is only an average and really only applies to women with a regular 28-day menstrual cycle. A woman who has a shorter cycle, say three weeks, will have

3	17/24	18/25	19/26	20/27	21/28	22/29	23/30	24/31	25/1	26/2	27/3	28/4	29/5	30/6	31/7
3	17/24	18/25	19/26	20/27	21/28	22/29	23/30	24/1	25/2	26/3	27/4	28/5			
1	17/22	18/23	19/24	20/25	21/26	22/27	23/28	24/29	25/30	26/31	27/1	28/2	29/3	30/4	31/5
1	17/22	18/23	19/24	20/25	21/26	22/27	23/28	24/29	25/30	26/31	27/1	28/2	29/3	30/4	
0	17/21	18/22	19/23	20/24	21/25	22/26	23/27	24/28	25/1	26/2	27/3	28/4	29/5	30/6	31/7
6/3	17/24	18/25	19/26	20/27	21/28	22/29	23/30	24/31	25/1	26/2	27/3	28/4	29/5	30/6	
6/2	17/23	18/24	19/25	20/26	21/27	22/28	23/29	24/30	25/1	26/2	27/3	28/4	29/5	30/6	31/7
6/3	17/24	18/25	19/26	20/27	21/28	22/29	23/30	24/31	25/1	26/2	27/3	28/4	29/5	30/6	31/7
6/3	17/24	18/25	19/26	20/27	21/28	22/29	23/30	24/1	25/2	26/3	27/4	28/5	29/6	30/7	
6/3	17/24	18/25	19/26	20/27	21/28	22/29	23/30	24/31	25/1	26/2	27/3	28/4	29/5	30/6	31/7
6/3	17/24	18/25	19/26	20/27	21/28	22/29	23/30	24/31	25/1	26/2	27/3	28/4	29/5	30/6	
6/2	17/23	18/24	19/25	20/26	21/27	22/28	23/29	24/30	25/1	26/2	27/3	28/4	29/5	30/6	31/7

ovulated earlier and will therefore probably deliver a week earlier. Her EDD will be 6 March. On the other hand, a woman who has a longer menstrual cycle, say five weeks, may be given a due date of 20 March to allow for ovulation taking place a week later. However, 85% of women deliver within two days of their EDD.

If your pattern of menstruation is irregular and/or you are unclear as to the date of your last period, other methods of determining a due date may be used by the doctor when you go for your first ante-natal visit, for instance, a pelvic examination to estimate the size of the uterus, or an ultrasound scan at a later date, but if the scan date and the EDD vary by less than a month, believe the EDD. If the scan date varies by more than a month from the EDD, believe the scan date. Always bear in mind that these dates are approximations. The length of a pregnancy is determined by hormones released by the placenta, and the placenta grows from the fertilized egg, not the mother.

The developing baby

The baby's life actually begins the moment the nuclei of the egg and the sperm fuse to form the first cell of the embryo. This cell then divides and redivides until it has about 64 cells in a cluster which is called a morula (Latin for mulberry).

The cells continue to multiply and the morula develops a hollow centre filled with fluid (the blastocyst). In the blastocyst the cells split into two parts one of which forms the embryo itself, the other the placenta and amniotic sac (the bag of fluid in which the baby grows).

By the time that menstruation would normally be due, about two weeks after fertilization of the egg, the blastocyst is well embedded in the wall of the uterus. The group of placental cells produce many villi, tiny roots that go into the endometrium (the uterus lining) to make contact with its blood vessels in search of oxygen and nutrients. These villi later develop into the true placenta supplying all the needs of the fetus (and taking away all the waste products that the developing life produces) until he or she is born.

For the first eight weeks of its life (when it is usually referred to as the embryo) the baby grows at an incredible rate developing from a cluster of cells to a complex organism with a brain, nervous system, skeleton, heart, lungs and other organs. During the rest of the pregnancy these vital structures not only grow but develop in complexity and sophistication until the baby is fully mature (at about 40 weeks, 280 days).

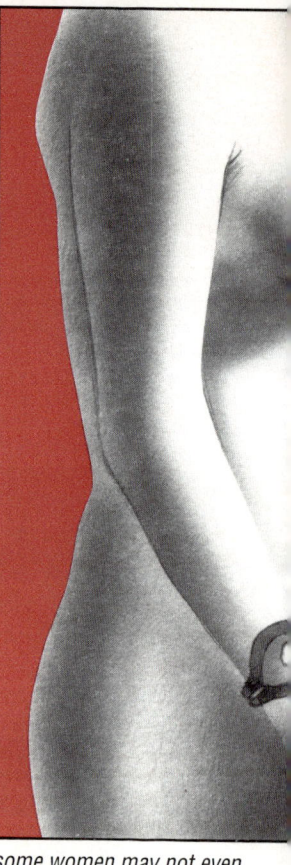

A calendar of development

When we refer to six weeks of pregnancy we are calculating from the first day of the last menstrual period. The embryo is actually four weeks old.

Baby at six weeks
Not recognizable as a human being, the embryo is 1.25 cm long with a reptilian head and a little tail and looks more like a tadpole. You can just see the buds of arms and legs. Nevertheless it already has the beginnings of a nervous system and blood vessels. The placenta has increased in size as has the uterus.

Changes in your body
You will probably experience some of the different symptoms of early pregnancy described earlier although some women may not even have noticed they are pregnant.

Baby at eight weeks
The embryo has grown to 2.5 cm and is more human in appearance though the head is still larger than the body. Limbs, even fingers, toes, eyes and ears are formed. The internal organs are in place, the stomach and kidney are in

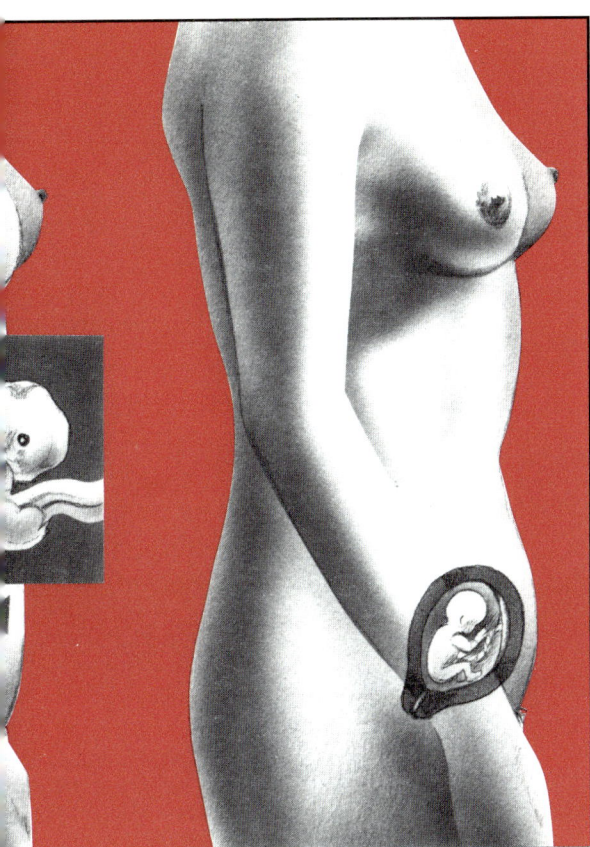

limb movements. It swallows the fluid from the amniotic sac and passes urine back into it. The blood moving round the lungs moves in regular bursts.

Changes in your body

Confident in your pregnancy, you should be feeling more settled and may be able to feel the uterus rising up out of your pelvis. Fatigue, nausea and vomiting usually lessen and stop at around this time. Your heart and lungs have to work much harder than before but you will not be aware of this.

Baby at 16 weeks

The fetus's heart is beating strongly and the muscles are becoming active so much so that you can sometimes feel its movements. In a first pregnancy this may not be noticeable until later, 18-20 weeks, because you will not be familiar with the fluttering feeling that early movements produce.

The fetus is about 18 cms long and weighs 100 g. The head is still rather large but the body length is growing fast. The reproductive organs are developing and it is possible at about this stage to tell what sex your baby will be.

Changes in your body

Most noticeable will be the quickening, the fluttery feeling

action and the heart is beating. The lungs, however, still form a solid mass.

Changes in your body

One important change is connected with your blood pressure in early pregnancy. It falls, and this can lead to light-headedness and even fainting especially if you have to stand for any length of time.

Baby at 12 weeks

Nine centimetres long and weighing about 15 g the fetus is gaining details such as finger and toe nails as well as showing signs of external genitalia. The head is still overlarge compared to the body but a face is clearly visible. The fetus's muscle and nerve coordination is improving fast and this can be seen in the more controlled inside you as the fetus stirs. The uterus can easily be felt, now reaching halfway from your navel and bulging out a bit. You are beginning to look pregnant.

The baby at 20 weeks
The fetus is growing at a tremendous rate, twisting and turning around freely in the amniotic sac - it is 25 cm long and weighs about 325 g.

Although he or she now looks human, the skin is covered with a fine hair known as lanugo. A baby is sometimes born with some of this still on but loses it very soon. The teeth are forming in the jawbone.

Changes in your body
You feel the baby stretching and kicking and are aware of very little movement at all when the baby rests. The uterus is up to the level of your navel.

During mid-pregnancy women usually feel on top form and it shows in the condition of the skin which benefits from the high hormone levels and increased blood circulation. Hair, on the other hand, may get drier if normally dry, greasier if greasy. However, you loose less than the average 100 hairs a day from your head during pregnancy, so your hair is thicker with more body.

Baby at 24 weeks
Wrinkled and covered in down, the fetus is scrawny but near fully formed although the lungs could still not maintain

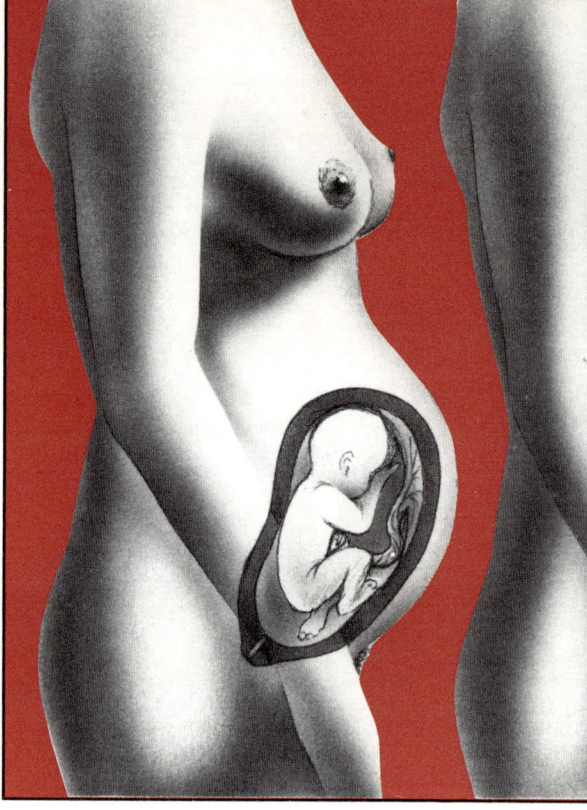

life should it be born this early. Some babies at this stage of pregnancy have survived outside the womb but only with expert care. The fetus measures about 32 cm and weighs about 650 g.

Changes in your body
Most women feel well at this stage, sleeping well and suffering only from a little backache as they begin to balance the weight of the belly. This is probably the period of your most rapid weight gain. Your heart and lungs are working hard doing

approximately 50% more work than before you were pregnant. You may find you sweat more, but you will also feel the cold less.

Baby at 28 weeks
Still thin, the fetus is 38 cm long and weighs 1000 g. The body is covered in the creamy vernix caseosa which is still there at birth and which protects the baby's skin from the amniotic fluid. The eyes can open and if the baby was born early, there would be about a 25% chance of survival because the lungs are

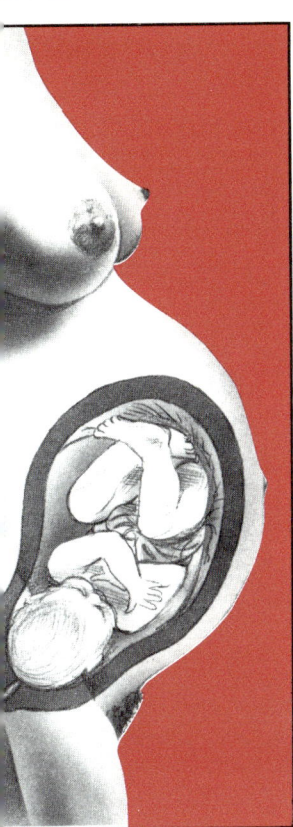

half a minute before relaxing again. These are known as Braxton Hicks contractions and are perfectly normal. Stretch marks may appear during this time.

Baby at 32 weeks

The fetus is still rather wrinkled but putting on fat fast, weighing about 1750 g and measuring 43 cms long. The lungs are usually well enough developed for a baby born at this stage to live, though still only with expert care. It is thought that by now the fetus can hear loud noises and respond to them with increased activity. It can certainly get the hiccups.

Changes in your body

Fatigue creeps up again as you near the end of pregnancy, not only from the weight you carry but also from an increase in the progesterone in your blood. This increased production helps to prevent premature labour by stifling the contractions.

During this stage you may find that ankles and feet swell, particularly at the end of the day. The linea nigra can be seen running down the abdomen from your navel which sticks out because of the increased size of the developing uterus.

Baby at 36 weeks

The baby has put on weight and plumped out (to 2.5 kg) losing the scrawny look as fat is deposited under the skin to provide energy and help to

regulate body heat after birth. Most babies born at this stage of maturity survive.

Changes in your body

Tired, suffering from backache and heartburn and sometimes unable to concentrate or to sleep comfortably, most women begin from now on to wish it were all over. However, one plus is the lightening which occurs about this time in women having their first baby. The baby's head descends into the pelvic cavity and gives you the feeling of a bit more breathing space for a short while.

Baby at 40 weeks

About 50 cm long and weighing an average of 3.4 kg your full-term baby is ready to live its own life. Its skin is smooth and greasy, sometimes still with a little lanugo down. The eyes are open. The genitals are fully formed and in a male child the testicles have descended into the scrotum. Movement will have slowed down (there is less room of course) as has growth rate. The placenta has stopped growing too.

Changes in your body

The uterus reaches right up to your ribs and contractions continue, almost unnoticed, until they become labour pains. By now you will be impatient for the baby to arrive, if it has not done so already. In fact, 80% of babies arrive within ten days either way of the full 40 weeks.

still at a very early stage of development.

Changes in your body

The uterus is well up above the level of the navel now and as the body responds to the muscle-relaxing hormones released by the placenta in preparation for birth many women suffer from heartburn and constipation.

You may notice among other movements within the uterus, slight painless contractions of the uterus itself as the whole of your stomach hardens for about

Childbirth

The reliable signs of labour:
• *Regular and painful contractions that may start as no more than 'lower backache' or 'like period pains', lasting initially about 30 seconds and coming every 15-20 minutes. It is usually advised that if you are having regular contractions about every 10 minutes then you should contact your hospital or midwife.*
• *A 'show'. This means the loss, often when you go to the toilet, of the plug of bloodstained mucus that has blocked the cervical canal throughout the pregnancy and has now been loosened as the cervix begins to dilate.*
• *The waters breaking. This may be a gush of liquid as dramatic as the old expression makes it sound - again sometimes when you visit the toilet, and sometimes coming together with the 'show' - or it may be no more than a dribble that you find you can't control. It is caused by the membranes of the amniotic sac rupturing and you should definitely phone the hospital or your midwife when it happens as labour usually follows within a few hours. Often, though, a sudden and unexpected bout of urinary incontinence can mimic it. This is because pressure from the baby's head distorts the usual feelings of wanting to pass urine.*

In the last few weeks of pregnancy the baby settles into what will be its final position; if it is a first birth the head may already be 'engaged' in the pelvis. Now the Braxton Hicks contractions - regular tightenings of the uterus that occur throughout pregnancy, usually without being noticed - become more severe and may lead you to suppose that labour has actually begun. This is known as 'false labour' and it is quite common for expectant mothers to be admitted to hospital overnight only to be discharged when the (irregular) contractions lessen in intensity and fade away completely.

The three stages of labour

Labour itself is commonly divided into three stages: from the onset of labour to full dilation of the cervix; from this point to delivery of the baby; delivery of the placenta (afterbirth).

First stage

No one really knows what triggers off the onset of labour at a particular point in time but it usually starts with a quiet phase lasting roughly nine hours in a first birth, four hours in others. During this time the contractions are not harsh and occur at long intervals, only gradually becoming stronger and more frequent. With each contraction the uterus muscles retract a little, pulling on the cervix and gradually shortening its 'cuff' where it projects into the vagina. This process is known as cervical effacement, or more descriptively, the 'taking up of the cervix', and it is followed by a stage where each further contraction pulling on the cervix gradually opens it - dilates it is the term used - to its full extent. The extent of dilation is measured in finger-breadths or centimetres and this quiet phase comes to an end as the diameter of the cervix reaches two to three finger-breadths (4-5 cm).

Transitional stage

After this point the contractions get much stronger and come with less of an interval between them. The baby moves further down into the pelvis, pressing on the bladder and back-passage, and you may begin to want very much to push it out. You have to resist this urge however until the cervix is fully dilated, at 8 cm, or the baby's head will not be able to pass through.

It is during this stage that you may need to call upon the techniques you have learned to cope with the pain as well as to prevent yourself from pushing. You may also find you want some sort of pain-relief.

The transitional stage usually lasts from 30 minutes to an hour.

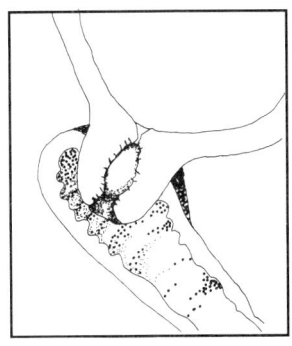

Second stage
When the cervix is fully dilated labour moves into the second stage when you have to do more than try to relax and endure and work begins in earnest.

This stage often begins with the waters breaking, if they have not done so already. You really have an irresistible urge to push now and as you do the baby moves down the newly created passageway, turning its head from facing into your hip to facing your back. As you push, holding your breath and bearing down with each powerful contraction, the baby's head gradually appears in the vulval opening, retreats then reappears, a little bit more being visible each time.

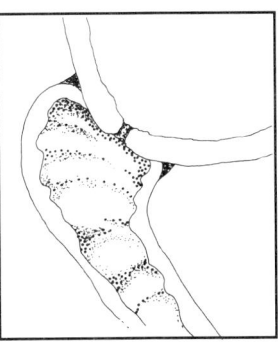

Then there is the 'crowning of the head' as it bulges out and finally the head is delivered, forehead first, and turns back round to face your hip again so that its shoulders and body slip out without any trouble with the next contractions. You will be asked to stop bearing down while the head is actually delivered so that it can come out slowly and gently rather than bursting out, tearing you as it comes.

Before the cervix begins to dilate, it points down into the vagina (top). As the contractions become stronger, the cervix becomes shorter and shorter until it no longer points down into the vagina (below), and the opening enlarges. Once the cervix is fully dilated, the second stage of labour has begun.

This second stage lasts on average an hour with first births and may be as short as 15 or 20 minutes with subsequent ones.

Third stage
This involves the delivery of the placenta or afterbirth which will have become detached from the uterus wall

Breastfeeding and bottle-feeding

An alert baby will search for the nipple within minutes of birth and you can stimulate this 'rooting reflex' by touching his cheek gently with your breast, the nipple close to the corner of the baby's mouth.

• Colostrum

Colostrum is produced by the breasts for the first couple of days following the birth. It is rich in protein, vitamins and minerals and low in sugar and fat. It also serves as a laxative to clear the baby's bowels of accumulated meconium and to give the baby something to keep going until the milk comes in - he or she has to continue sucking for this to be produced at all.

• Breast milk

Breast milk is the ideal baby food (and drink) containing a well-balanced supply of nutrients, enzymes, hormones and antibodies to promote good health and protect the baby from infection. As a consequence breastfed babies are far less likely to be overweight (as babies and thus as children and adults) or to suffer from illnesses from gastro-enteritis to measles and chest infections.
Breast milk is always available at the right temperature in the right quantity (supply follows demand) and it may even serve to influence your baby's

with the birth of the baby and which further, less painful, contractions eventually expel. Expulsion is sometimes aided by gentle pulling on the umbilical cord or by the action of a synthetic hormone drug injected into the mother as soon as the baby is delivered. It is important that the whole of the placenta comes out or it can lead to hemorrhaging later on.

After the birth

It is sometimes said that putting your baby straight to the breast should be considered as the fourth stage of labour because suckling causes the release of the hormone oxytocin which helps the uterus to shrink back more rapidly to its normal size, thus both lessening any bleeding and returning your body sooner to its pre-pregnancy weight and shape.

First feeding

For the first two to three days after the birth the breasts give not milk but colostrum, a yellowish high-protein fluid (this often leaks out from the nipples even before the birth), and it is this that keeps the baby going until the milk 'comes in' on about the third day.

The breasts don't begin to produce milk at all until the baby is actually born. Milk production is prompted by the action of a hormone, prolactin, which is secreted by the pituitary gland, but during pregnancy the high level of the sex hormones estrogen and progesterone prevents the prolactin from acting. When the level of these sex hormones drops upon birth (they are produced by the placenta), the milk-producing cells of the alveoli inside the breasts get to work.

The prolactin was itself produced in the beginning in response to messages to the pituitary from the brain, and once the baby begins to take the milk the actual suckling does the job of prompting the production of yet more prolactin and thus more milk.

The oxytocin mentioned earlier as valuable in restoring the uterus to its previous shape also serves to trigger the milk 'let-down' reflex whereby the milk inside the breasts is forced out down the milk ducts ready for feeding. Here again, it is a message from the brain prompted by the suckling, or even by hearing your baby cry and wanting to feed him, that prompts the pituitary to produce the oxytocin.

Inside the uterus

Within the uterus the baby floats in the clear amniotic fluid, attached by the umbilical cord to the placenta which is in turn attached to the lining of the uterus.

The placenta

In the very early days of the pregnancy the placental cells completely surround the new embryo, their little 'fingers', or villi, implanted in the lining of the uterus (the endometrium). Later, around the twelfth week, the outer villi die off, those that remain being grouped in a circular area on the uterus wall. After the fourteenth week or so this becomes the placenta proper which then proceeds to grow as the baby grows.

It is fully developed by the fourth month of pregnancy, being about the same size as the baby at this point and 7.5 cm in diameter. At full term it is more like 18-20 cm in diameter and weighs about 0.5 kg. It does not however continue to grow throughout the pregnancy but reaches a peak at about the thirty-fourth week after which it begins, very slowly, to degenerate though it is normally still efficient even when a pregnancy runs over term (becoming overdue) into 42 weeks.

Doctors worry about the placenta not functioning adequately if the baby is overdue and may do checks on this just in case, especially with older mothers, the over thirty-five-year-olds.

The villi are made up of a network of fine, tiny blood vessels enclosed in a membrane lined with placental cells. These hundreds of villi (which have an enormous surface area) project into a sort of lake of blood made by the placenta in the lining of the uterus. From this the villi absorb oxygen and nutrients for the baby while discharging into the lake the baby's carbon dioxide and other waste

future health, the low cholesterol and high unpolysaturates level protecting against heart disease as an adult. And of course breastfeeding is cheap. The mother does require extra calories but many of these have been laid down during pregnancy in the extra weight a woman carries. Breastfeeding is practical, involving no mixing or sterilizing, and no equipment to carry or remember when you go out! It helps you to lose weight more quickly after the birth and finally, it is above all deeply satisfying and pleasurable to both parties.

• Bottlefeeding

On the other hand, if you can't breastfeed for any reason (for example, if your baby is premature and too small to suck), content yourself with the fact that bottlefed babies grow up perfectly strong and healthy. But do make sure you give your baby the same quality of cuddling closeness during the feeds as he or she would have naturally if breastfeeding.

The great advantage of bottlefeeding is that your partner can share much more in the feeding routine and the wonderful experience of cuddling and bonding as the baby feeds.

products (to be carried away into the mother's blood-stream and dealt with by her body mechanisms). The nutrients absorbed in this way include everything the baby needs from carbohydrates, vitamins and protein to essential elements such as iron and calcium - the baby gets first pick of what is available.

In spite of this closeness, the two circulations are at all times kept separate by the placental cells through which everything has to pass, but they act as a partial filter only. Apart from necessary food and waste other substances can also cross·the placenta, most importantly some antibodies made by the mother in response to germs; these give the baby immunity to the illnesses they cause when it is born and for some time after.

Unfortunately, although it was once believed that the placenta filtered out everything that might harm the baby, substances that may be damaging to the baby can also cross the placenta, for instance drugs and alcohol. This is especially significant in early pregnancy while the embryo is still being formed because of the danger of deformities: the rubella (German measles) virus falls into this category.

It is thought that all these substances may take as little as an hour to pass from the mother's blood circulation to that of the baby.

The umbilical cord

The tiny blood vessels of the villi eventually join into the two fetal arteries and the fetal vein. These run from the centre of the placenta to the navel (umbilicus) of the baby within the umbilical cord, a transparent membrane sheath round the spiralling blood vessels. Filled with a greeny blue jelly the umbilical cord grows as the baby does, and by the time of the baby's birth is as thick as a finger and long enough for the baby to be held by the mother while the placenta is still attached to the uterus wall.

The amniotic sac and fluid

The amniotic sac is made up of two layers of membrane. The thin outer layer is in one piece with the sheath of the umbilical cord while the inner layer contains the amniotic fluid in which the baby floats. Together they provide a strong but flexible protective 'balloon' in which the baby can live safely and even exercise.

The fluid, sometimes referred to as the liquor or the waters, is formed early in the development of the embryo and contains nutrients important for the baby's growth; its exact make-up varies as the pregnancy progresses, for instance in later stages when the baby passes urine into the fluid.

The volume of fluid also varies; in the beginning it is high compared to the size of the baby which helps extend the uterus to make room for the baby. Later the amount of fluid increases more slowly until in the last month there is barely enough for the baby to move about in which is why the baby appears to move less vigorously as the pregnancy progresses. By the birth there is an average of 800 ml only.

The fluid not only provides a way for the baby to excrete waste, including urine, but also allows the baby to 'practise' swallowing and inhaling (though the lungs do not expand) in preparation for birth.

Finally the amniotic sac provides a sterile and cushioning environment, always at a constant temperature, for the baby to develop in. It remains whole until the onset of or during labour and is afterwards expelled as part of the afterbirth together with the placenta and umbilical cord. It is known, though rare, for the baby's head to be delivered with the sac membrane still intact - 'in a caul' - a sign of good luck in many cultures.

The blood circulation

The fetal heart starts to beat by about the seventh week of pregnancy and pumps the blood round its body at between 110 and 170 beats per minute, depending on whether the fetus is active or not. This averages out at 140 beats per minute which is double the rate of the mother's heart (as mentioned above the two blood circulations should never mingle).

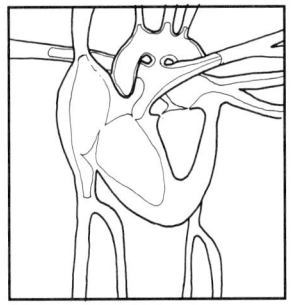

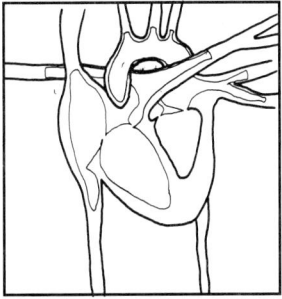

Because the fetus obtains its oxygen from its mother's blood via the placenta, not from the lungs, the fetal blood doesn't pass through its lungs at all but goes through an opening within the heart direct to the rest of its body (top). This opening, the foramen ovale, closes at birth (below) as the baby's lungs expand for the first time and the blood begins to pass through them on its journey round the body.

Staying healthy

Before conception

Routine ante-natal care, regular check-ups and attention paid to the everyday well-being of the mother and her baby during pregnancy, is a relatively recent concept going back only 40 or 50 years. Today's mothers tend to take it for granted and its value in promoting both her and the baby's health is well recognized.

Today the quest for optimum health and safety in pregnancy and childbirth is causing us to look even further back, to the time before conception, and analyze factors such as diet and exercise as well as working and living environment and the possible pollutants we may come into contact with. It may be difficult to believe that these factors can have an effect on a pregnancy that has not even begun, but research has proved strong links between a tendency to miscarriage or low weight at birth and the absorption of certain substances by the mother, or less often the father.

If what you take into your body can have such a powerful effect on your baby, especially in the very early days which is when you are most likely to be unaware you are pregnant at all, it surely makes sense if you are trying to get pregnant or even just thinking about it to take a good look at your diet and lifestyle. The Chinese are perhaps recognizing the importance of the time the baby spends in the womb when they take him to be one year old at birth!

For discussion and support you may like to join one of the self-help groups formed for this purpose or attend a special pre-conceptual clinic. Your doctor should also be willing to give you advice and perhaps a general health check-up including a blood test to check your hemoglobin (to make sure you are not anemic) and to confirm that you are immune to rubella (German measles). Avoid becoming obsessive, looking for problems and making yourself over-anxious (certainly no way to get pregnant). Take a positive approach and do not fret over things that cannot be altered, for example, if you have inadvertently received an X-ray before you realized you were pregnant.

Contraception

You want your body to be running naturally, not artificially interfered with when you conceive. If you have an IUD (coil) fitted, have this removed in good time and let your menstrual periods resume their natural flow and frequency. Use a barrier method such as a condom (sheath) or diaphragm instead for two or three months.

If you are on the Pill, discontinue taking this and, again, allow three menstrual cycles to complete before you allow yourself to become pregnant. This will restore your periods to their natural rhythm making it easier to date the conception and thus work out your due date.

Diet

During the period before conception you should get yourself into tip-top condition in terms of nutrition so that you can provide a thoroughly healthy environment for the new embryo to develop in. Research has shown, for example, that good nutrition can affect the way the uterus develops during pregnancy, which in turn may determine its efficiency in labour.

Good nutrition means eating sensibly with a full awareness of the importance of variety in your diet rather than just quantity - no 'eating for two'. You need carbohydrates and fat for energy (in early pregnancy you may be resting but you have the equivalent of someone running furiously on the spot inside you), protein for the formation of body tissue, and vitamins and minerals to help in the chemical processes of the body.

A recent study has shown that mothers whose intake of these essential nutrients is below recommended levels tend to produce babies of lower than average birth weight. A baby of lower than average weight at birth is not inevitably in bad shape either physically or mentally, but definite links have been established between low birth weight and slow physical and mental development. Low birth weight can also mean that a new baby is not as strong and has fewer resources to call upon should other health problems arise.

Finally, in support of the pre-conception care lobby, statistics from the dreadful 'hunger winter' in Holland in 1944 indicate that the incidence of perinatal mortality, stillbirths and underweight babies was greater among women who conceived at this time than among those who gave birth during this time.

Exercise

Be positive again. Get your body into trim with regular, not-too-arduous exercise. Do not decide to take up skiing or horse riding at this point, but establish a pattern of exercise that you can go on with into pregnancy, even if you have to slow down a bit later on. Swimming is probably the most relaxing complete form of exercise for the mother-to-be and may be indulged in, moreover, right to the end of the pregnancy.

Damaging substances

Drugs

The shock of the thalidomide babies made everyone all too aware of how readily medicinal drugs can cross the placenta into the baby and affect it dreadfully. Only a few such drugs have been proved definitely to be harmful but there is really no way of knowing in advance whether any particular drug will damage a baby, especially when even a high-risk drug may not affect every baby whose mother has taken it.

If you are considering becoming pregnant it is probably better simply to avoid all painkillers, antacids and tranquillizers, hay fever treatments, even the humble aspirin, altogether. Ask the doctor for advice if you need antibiotics or if, when pregnant, you want anti-nausea tablets and make sure he or she knows you are or are trying to become pregnant if they are prescribed. For example, particular types of antibiotics can permanently discolour the developing teeth of the baby you are carrying, but others will not and an alternative can be prescribed.

This is especially important in the first three months when the cells of the embryo are dividing at their fastest. It should also be borne in mind later when you are

• **Illegal drugs**
All of the illegal drugs you are likely to come across are potentially or absolutely damaging to a baby so do not touch them.

• **Regular medication**
Let your doctor know you are trying or intending to conceive so that you can check over continuation of any regular medication. Some prescriptions may have to be modified.

breastfeeding as some drugs will cross into your milk.

Tobacco

A whole string of problems are associated with babies of smokers; there is no doubt at all that smoking cigarettes is seriously damaging - before conception as well as during pregnancy and after the birth.

There is a direct link between smoking and a reduction in the number of cells produced in both the body and the brain of a fetus; nicotine causes a reduction in the blood supply to the fetus; the high level of carbon monoxide in a smoker's blood reduces the amount of oxygen it can carry to the fetus and so on. The end result is babies of lower than average birth weight who are more likely to miscarry or die soon after birth and are more often born prematurely.

The risks of congenital abnormality brought on by smoking apply not only to those who smoke during pregnancy but also to those who smoke when the baby is conceived. Children of heavy smoking fathers may be twice as likely to suffer from some malformation. Research also shows that smokers both male and female are more likely to be infertile or take longer to conceive.

If you smoke, give it up, or at the very least cut right down. However, remember that there is no safe level of smoking.

Alcohol

This has only fairly recently been linked to presenting real risk to the unborn child, and can sometimes affect physical and/or mental development. Damage done may range from a low birth weight and lower than average intelligence to abnormal facial and limb formation, and it may occur as a result of drinking at any point during pregnancy, but especially between six and twelve weeks.

Obviously regular, heavy drinking is to blame in most cases but it is thought that even one bout of heavy drinking or as little as two drinks each day may sometimes lead to problems (though these may be slight and not necessarily visible or obvious).

Finally, not only is alcohol a poison in itself but it also acts negatively as an anti-nutrient, affecting the good absorption of nutrients, such as the absorption of zinc, which is greatly needed by the body in pregnancy. So, avoid more than the occasional drink. Many women now choose to forgo alcohol completely while they are pregnant - and indeed in the period immediately before lest their drinking even pre-conception have an effect.

Rubella

If you are planning to become pregnant you should certainly check with your doctor as to whether you are immune to rubella (German measles). It is very likely that you will have had the disease or been vaccinated against it in childhood or even as an adult but don't rely on your mother's 'Yes, I think so' when you ask her - have a blood test. If no rubella antibodies are present in your blood you will have to be vaccinated and then wait for three months before you attempt to become pregnant. (Most girls are now vaccinated routinely before they are thirteen.)

The trouble is that although German measles is only a mild disease with a slight rash and perhaps a high temperature, the rubella virus is one of the few organisms that can cross the placenta and infect the fetus directly. Should this happen during the first 12 weeks of pregnancy it is likely to seriously damage the fetal organs causing deafness, blindness and abnormalities of the heart.

If you are already pregnant and have not had German measles take care to avoid anyone who may have it or have been in contact with it. If you suspect that you have come into contact with rubella it may be possible to prevent the disease developing by having an injection of gamma globulin; ask your doctor at once. If you actually develop the disease you must also let the doctor know immediately, especially if this happens in the first 12 weeks.

Should a diagnosis of rubella be confirmed by the presence in your blood of antibodies that were not there before, you may wish to consider having a termination because of the high risk of serious damage involved. This is obviously a very personal matter.

If you are already immune there is nothing to fear from contact with the disease at all. This is why it is best to sort the matter out before you get pregnant in the first place.

X-rays

The dose of radiation in a medical X-ray being given for ordinary diagnostic purposes is very low but there seems still to be disagreement over whether this is likely to harm significantly a developing embryo or fetus. Some doctors say no, but others claim that X-rays sometimes upset the genes in the chromosomes within both male and female reproductive organs, which may ultimately lead to abnormalities in a later generation. Also, some doctors believe that exposure of the fetus to X-rays may be linked to some childhood leukaemia.

Radiology departments and dentists' surgeries usually display signs telling you to inform the technician if you are or may be pregnant before you have an X-ray. Don't hesitate to do this even if you are not sure. They will protect your abdomen from the X-rays with a lead screen or apron. If an X-ray is required of your abdomen, pelvis or lower back for any reason, it may be recommended that you have them taken during the first ten days of your menstrual cycle to avoid any possibility of irradiating a fetus, although there is still some disagreement about this.

VDUs

Claims have been made recently that women working non-stop, every day at VDUs (visual display units of computers) are at increased risk of miscarrying when pregnant, and less likely to become pregnant in the first place, while doing this sort of work. If you are having trouble conceiving you may feel it worth your while changing your job to avoid this risk, but keep problems such as this in perspective. Remember that one in six couples have difficulty getting (one another) pregnant.

After conception

Vitamins

A good supply is essential to the baby's growth.

• Vitamin A is found in egg yolk, fish oils (especially cod liver oil), milk, butter and cheese, margarine, fresh fruit, spinach and tomatoes, brussels sprouts, beetroot and carrots.

• Vitamin B_1 is present in beans, peas, nuts and wheat (can be taken as wheatgerm oil), brown rice, eggs, offal and fish oils.

• Vitamin B_2 is again present in offal and in meat, fish and shellfish, milk, cheese and cream, nuts, yeast, peas and beans.

• Vitamin B_{12}, known also as riboflavin, is found in animal products.

• Vitamin C is found in fresh fruit and vegetables and milk.

• Vitamin D is found in fish oils and animal fats, cheese, butter, milk and eggs but is made by the skin if it is exposed to ultraviolet light in the sunshine.

Once you know you are pregnant look after yourself. This means eating and drinking sensibly, getting enough of both rest and exercise and preparing yourself mentally and in practical ways for the arrival of your baby. But it also means continuing with other aspects of your life that are important to you, such as sex, work, your hobbies and social life. Lead a healthy life with full awareness of your pregnancy but don't become obsessed by it to the exclusion of all else - and remember this is a precious time when you can do things you won't be able to later!

Eating sensibly

Probably the most important thing is to eat a well-balanced diet containing a wide range of foods. That way you can be sure of gaining all the nutrients you and the baby need without constantly consulting charts and making yourself over-anxious. However, it can be helpful to know which foods fall into each of the categories that fulfil a different nutritional need, so that for instance you can substitute a chunk of cheese for the recommended daily intake of milk (fat, protein and calcium) or dried apricots and beans for iron-rich meat such as liver.

Protein

Eat meat, including offal, fish and shellfish, eggs, cheese and milk. Peas, beans, lentils, seeds, and nuts also contain protein. Your protein requirement increases by about 50%.

Carbohydrate

Go easy on foods containing flour or sugar which are high in carbohydrate. They include bread, cereals, potatoes, rice, pasta, cakes and pastries, honey, jam, syrup and chocolate - and all sweets.

Fats

Moderate amounts of fat are needed but remember they tend to be high in calorie content. They include milk, cream and cheese, butter and mayonnaise, cooking oils and fats and of course the fat on meat, especially bacon.

Fluids and fibre

Keep your digestive system working well by drinking plenty of liquids. Water is probably best, for the benefit of the kidneys. Eat plenty of roughage, fibrous foods such as wholemeal bread, brown rice, raw fruit and vegetables, peas and beans.

Salt

A high intake of sodium is associated with a raised blood pressure, something that should definitely be avoided during pregnancy. Most of our sodium comes from table salt, although flavour enhancers such as monosodium glutamate and raising agents such as sodium bicarbonate are also high in sodium. In fact in Europe we take in 100 times more salt than we need, but only 30% of this comes from the salt we add ourselves to food. The rest is hidden in manufactured and processed food.

During pregnancy you must keep your salt intake down as much as possible. The simplest way to do this is to avoid eating processed and manufactured foods as well as cutting out salt in your cooking. You may find food tastes a little bland at first, but your palate will quickly adjust.

Weight gain

The weight you put on in pregnancy is not just that of the actual baby (plus placenta and amniotic fluid) but is also due to your increased blood circulation and breast and uterus size as well as the fat laid down in your body in preparation for breastfeeding. Towards the end of pregnancy retained fluid will account for some of this extra weight.

Weight gain varies according to the size you are initially, whether you suffer from morning sickness (causing weight loss), your metabolism and lifestyle, as well as what you eat - and how much of it! Similarly, some women put on a lot of weight in the first months then find weight gain levels off while others increase in weight gradually throughout the 40 weeks.

A vegetarian diet

It may not be a good idea to become vegetarian during pregnancy as it can take a while to work out how to achieve the same sort of balanced diet as you are used to without eating meat. If you are already vegetarian, however, there should not be any problem though you should be extra aware of which plant foods provide you with iron and eat plenty of them.

In the same way vegans must ensure an adequate intake of calcium, vitamin D and vitamin B_{12}, all of which non-vegans get from dairy products. Also they will need to keep taking supplementary vitamin B_{12} as this comes only from animal products.

Resting
Make the most of the opportunities that come your way: sit where you would normally stand and lie down if you can or put your feet up when you would normally sit down. Also use simple relaxation techniques such as the following.
• Settle yourself comfortably.
• Take a deep breath, hold it for a few seconds then breathe out deeply, relaxing all your muscles at the same time.
• Check over your whole body bit by bit until you feel each part is completely relaxed.
• Empty your mind of everything and try to breathe slowly and regularly.

Most commonly, the period of rapid weight gain is between 24 and 32 weeks and loss in weight very often occurs after the 38th week. A good rule of thumb is to keep weight gain down to half a stone for each trimester (each three months) or half a pound a week, making you one and a half stone heavier when you go into labour.

Resting

Get as much rest as you can. Different women need different amounts of sleep but ideally you should aim for eight hours at night and two hours in the afternoon. This is not always possible of course, especially if you have a job or if you have other children to look after. However, even half-an-hour with your feet up on the desk or a brief lie-down on the bed is better than nothing - and toddlers who think they are too grown-up for an afternoon sleep can often be persuaded to join their mother in a short nap!

You may find the problem is that you get more sympathy and opportunity to rest when your bulge begins to show in the later stages whereas it is in the first three months that you feel absolutely devastated and long for bed - often before you have even told anyone you are pregnant. Women often feel at their most energetic during the middle three months.

At work

It is usual today for employed women to work normally through their pregnancy up to the point where state maternity benefits are available - at 29 weeks. This break-off point suits the majority although some will continue to work right up to the onset of labour without any sense of strain while others would be only too happy to stop work more or less as soon as pregnancy is confirmed.

A decision as to when you stop work will probably depend on several factors: how physically tiring or intellectually demanding the job is; how fit and well you are feeling; your childbearing history; and last but not least your financial situation. Whatever your position, while you are both pregnant and working make sure that the former gets priority over the latter. Don't exhaust yourself, don't take on projects you really can't cope with - don't be ashamed to slow down a bit.

If you decide to return to work after maternity leave, as an increasing number of women do, you may feel there is rather more pressure on you to keep going efficiently before you leave to have the baby. Again, don't let this bother you. Do what feels right to you: accept your condition and make sure your work colleagues do too.

Sex

As always with anything to do with sex there seem to be as many 'norms' for sex during pregnancy as there are pregnant women. One woman will enjoy sex more with the concern of getting or not getting pregnant gone or because higher levels of hormones circulating in her body have caused changes in her body such as a new fullness around her vagina. Her wish to express her love and happiness to her partner may also increase her sexual desire.

Another finds it irritating even to be touched - perhaps her nipples are over-sensitive and she feels tired and nauseous, or she may simply withdraw physically in a protective sort of way: she may worry about a miscarriage or damaging the baby.

To the question 'Can sexual intercourse harm the baby in any way?' the answer is usually 'No, but ...' The baby is cushioned in the uterus by the amniotic sac of fluid and sealed off by the cervix and mucous plug from the vagina; there is no risk of infection. Intercourse will not bring on a miscarriage nor orgasm (as maintained in the old wives' tale) bring on labour.

However, if you experience any bleeding, report this to your doctor who will have to check for placenta praevia and signs of miscarriage. It may be just a matter of spotting from ruptured blood vessels round the cervix in which case it may be suggested that you avoid deep penetration in lovemaking, but do check anyway.

If you have a history of miscarriage you will obviously want to be that much more careful and may be

37

advised to abstain from sex for the first three months until the pregnancy is established. (Similarly, in the last weeks, if you have previously had problems with premature labour.) It is also sometimes thought a good idea not to have sexual intercourse at those monthly intervals when you would have had your period, these being vulnerable times for the uterus.

If you are full of sexual desire go ahead and enjoy yourself - within limits as mentioned - but if you are one of the unlucky ones who fear that they have lost their libido altogether, don't worry. Many women feel like that but it does return, even if you have to wait until after you have finished breastfeeding, and sex can then be even better than before.

Ante-natal care

The introduction of regular ante-natal check-ups has made a huge difference to the number of mothers and babies who have emerged from pregnancy and childbirth in good health and spirits. Only 50 years ago the very concept of preventive medicine in pregnancy was unknown and the mother-to-be saw a doctor or midwife before labour began only if some complication arose, a complication, often, that could have been avoided. Statistics show moreover that the earlier a pregnant woman reports to her doctor for ante-natal care the more likely she is to enjoy a trouble-free pregnancy and give birth to a healthy baby.

Seeing the doctor

See your doctor as soon as you think you are pregnant so that he or she can confirm the pregnancy by checking your dates and perhaps doing a pregnancy test or internal examination. Once the pregnancy is confirmed you are eligible for free prescriptions and dental care, and maternity benefit where applicable.

This visit is an opportunity for you to discuss with your doctor the arrangements for your ante-natal care and eventual confinement. If you have strong feelings, for instance that you want a home birth, broach the subject now. Ask advice but don't be put off if you don't see eye to eye on the subject; you can usually transfer to another doctor in the practice or even to a neighbouring practice just for your obstetric care.

Where to go
There are usually several options open. You can book in at a local hospital and attend there for all your ante-natal care or you may prefer to see your doctor or a midwife for ante-natal care (many practices run special clinics) as well as having them look after your confinement at home. Shared care, where you check in at the hospital then see your doctor regularly up to the last few weeks when you return to the hospital, is a popular option: the doctor is usually closer and more convenient and you have the benefit of greater continuity for most of the pregnancy. If you attend a hospital clinic you rarely see the same staff - or indeed the other women attending - twice, and can begin to feel more of a number, even a nuisance, than a person.

The ante-natal clinic
Whichever option you choose your first visit will be very much the same. To build up as full a picture as possible of your health and circumstances you will be asked many questions from your shoe size (to help judge pelvic size) to your smoking habits and from menstrual history to the mental health of your parents. Some may seem irrelevant, or even offensive, such as asking your racial or national origin, but they can be vital - in the latter case, for instance, your blood will be tested for sickle cell anemia should you be of West African origin but for thalassemia if you are from certain parts of the Mediterranean or Middle East. Some subjects won't recur but other questions - and tests - will, at every visit. These will be monthly up to 28 weeks, two-weekly up to 36 weeks, then weekly until you go into labour.

Among things regularly checked are: your urine (for symptoms of diabetes, pre-eclampsia, kidney infection); your weight; your blood for blood grouping, to eliminate certain diseases and ensure you're not anemic; and your legs and hands (for varicose veins or swelling). Regular abdominal examinations check on the baby's growth and position and in later months the fetal heart beat will be listened for.

All this information goes down in your file but you also have a chance to ask questions and have your preferences as to whether you want pain relief, induced labour, etc recorded. Don't hesitate to voice any fears you have or to mention problems, however small they may seem.

Other tests

Alpha-feto protein test

Between 16 and 18 weeks a test is done to measure the amount of alpha-feto protein (AFP) in your blood. A high level at this stage may indicate abnormal development of the baby's brain or spinal cord (indicating anencephaly or spina bifida) but may just mean you are carrying twins or are further advanced in pregnancy than you thought. Any positive result is double-checked by means of ultrasound scanning, a further blood test and possibly amniocentesis.

Ultrasound

Most women now routinely have an ultrasound scan at about 16 weeks to check on the size and position of the fetus and this may be repeated, perhaps if the baby doesn't seem to be growing or if the AFP level is high and twins are suspected.

When you have a scan you are asked to lie on a couch with your abdomen uncovered (and your bladder full - this makes for a clearer picture). The technician will oil your abdomen and then smooth an ultrasonic sensor gently over it, repeatedly. This gives out and picks up sound waves which bounce back off the bones and tissues of the fetus and are converted into a clear image on a television screen. It can be a very exciting and moving moment when you see your baby for the first time. Sometimes you can buy a photo of the picture to keep.

Amniocentesis

This test is done under local anesthetic after an ultrasound scan has located the fetus and placenta in the uterus so as to avoid disturbing or damaging them. A sample of the amniotic fluid is then taken from the uterus by means of a needle inserted through the abdomen. It should be painless and takes only about ten minutes.

However, amniocentesis is not done routinely as there is a very small risk of provoking a miscarriage. It is usually offered when there is considered to be a greater risk of some chromosomal abnormality (such as Down's syndrome) or genetically linked disorders. Chromosomal tests are carried out on the embryo's shed skin cells revealing not only the sex of the fetus but also information about any possible inherited disorders which are carried on the sex chromosome, such as Down's syndrome or hemophilia .

Because the chances of giving birth to a Down's baby rise sharply after the age of 35 this test is usually available to women older than this. If you do have an amniocentesis for whatever reason you should think seriously in advance about your decision in the event of a positive result, that is, whether to terminate the pregnancy or not. Many women, opposed to termination whatever the reason, prefer not to embark down the road of amniocentesis from the start - others prefer to know.

Preparing for the birth

Use the months of your pregnancy to prepare yourself both physically and mentally for the birth of your baby (see pages 49-55). You will probably have to make up your mind at a fairly early stage where you want to give birth and your decision may well depend on your approach to childbirth. After reading as widely as you can and talking to other mothers and perhaps medical staff you will very likely find that you have plumped, albeit unconsciously, for one of the following.

Psychoprophylaxis

Also known as 'prepared' childbirth the techniques of psychoprophylaxis were introduced from Russia and seek to remove the pain from labour (a) by fully explaining the process of childbirth in the belief that it is fear that causes pain and ignorance that causes fear; and (b) by providing exercises and breathing techniques to help cope with it.

Today's active birth proponents have taken up these ideas but feel that it is also important that the mother learns how to relax properly in labour, accepting the contractions, and also suggest that she should be free to choose and change her position at any stage during labour.

This sort of approach is loosely termed 'natural' childbirth and you may well wish to follow it through by giving birth in the free and familiar surroundings of your own home - or alternatively under a Domino system (domiciliary in-and-out) where you give birth in hospital but return home promptly, attended before and after by your own midwife.

Positions for labour and birth

This is an area where there have been great changes in recent years as natural childbirth has spread its influence. It used to be the case that although moving around in the very early stages was acceptable, once labour was well established it was on to the bed. Today there is far more tolerance of different ways of coping with childbirth especially as to what position you want to adopt at any stage.

First stage
Standing
Many women are restless and want to move around, perhaps halting as a contraction starts and holding on to furniture or their partner for support (lean forward as you do this). Moving helps to get contractions going and may make their action more efficient - certainly it is a plus to have gravity assisting the baby's descent! Doing something rather than just lying still also distracts you from the discomfort of the contractions.

Sitting
If you are tired, sit on the edge of a (stable) chair leaning forwards, legs apart or sit astride a hard chair facing the back and using this for support.

Kneeling

Kneel on your haunches and lean with your arms and head on a large beanbag or cushioned chair seat. This is seen as a secure and comfortable position and is popular when the contractions are getting really strong; it is especially good for coping with the transitional stage. To reduce the intensity of contractions, go right down on all fours or even kneel with your elbows on the ground and bottom in the air - not a position recommended for those wearing the classic open-at-the-back hospital gown. Do this to counter gravity at the transitional stage, as you resist the urge to bear down.

Squatting

Squat on your heels and steady yourself by holding on to a firm chair seat or put a cushion under your heels or even pop a low stool under your bottom. This is the position in which your pelvis is most widely open. It is also one that intensifies contractions so it may be better if you stand up, using your partner as support, while you feel them.

Lying down

Of course you can just lie down (especially if you need a rest) on your side or front - with cushions keeping your head up and under your upper thigh too - not on your back because this impedes the flow of blood to the uterus. If you are on a bed, you can either lie on your side or lean back, almost upright, propped up on pillows.

If your back aches, leaning forward takes the pressure off it - whether you lean on your partner or a chair or go on all fours and lean forward, rocking to and fro. Gentle massage of the lower back can also help, or even a hot water bottle. Don't lie on your back.

Second stage

You may want still to move around and be free to do so, giving birth on the floor or on a mattress on the floor, but it is possible to give birth in various positions while on a standard hospital bed as well.

Squatting
You can either have someone sitting or kneeling in front of you to hold on to as you squat or someone sitting on a low stool behind you with his arms under your armpits. Or you can have one person on each side so you can put your arms round their shoulders. If you're on the floor they can give you additional support by taking some of your weight on their knees, but this position is also well suited to the hospital bed, with one supporter standing on either side. This position has the advantage of opening the pelvis to its greatest extent and also means that the baby can emerge almost unaided because you are so close to the ground/ bed. You may even be able to reach down and assist in the delivery yourself.

Standing squat
This involves your faithful supporter standing behind you with his arms under your armpits. He should lean slightly backwards with knees bent but back straight to take your weight. You have your feet well apart and set flat on the ground and as the contraction comes you allow your knees to bend; in between contractions stand or go on all fours to rest. Birth doesn't usually take long in this position but it won't be taken up until a fairly late stage, when the baby's head has already crowned.

Kneeling
The all fours position may be taken up either on the floor or on a bed but whichever it is make sure that you use a large bean bag or cushions to give good support to your upper body. Once they are used to this position most midwives like it as it gives them a good clear view of what is going on. It is one of the most commonly chosen positions.

Semi-upright
Propped up against cushions, this is the position usually taken up on the hospital bed. You draw up your legs now and hold them tight on either side of your abdomen as you labour, relaxing and letting your legs go in between.

On the side

The lateral position (left or right lateral, medically speaking) means on your side with one leg up - held by yourself or resting on the midwife's shoulder or on a stool. Lying on your side has the disadvantage that you don't take advantage of the effects of gravity at all - even less so than when semi-upright - but it does allow medical staff to see the baby coming out easily and to intervene quickly when they feel there is need, for instance to do an episiotomy. (This is also true of the semi-upright position and is the reason many doctors prefer these two positions above all.)

Analgesic-supported birth

An analgesic gives pain relief with full consciousness and several different types may be offered to you in labour.

A number of women also turn to the alternative therapies for pain relief during labour, and a guide to these is given in the tinted column of the next two pages.

Pethidine

Given in the form of an injection, pethidine relaxes and relieves anxiety, easing the pain of contractions. However, as it takes 15-20 minutes to have full effect and wears off after a few hours, more than one injection may be necessary and if it is given too near to delivery will not have time to act and will result in a very sleepy baby.

Gas and air

Inhaled through a self-held mask and the gas is given 'on demand'. This is valuable psychologically as much as anything else, giving you some feeling of being in control and helping yourself as a contraction approaches. Most inhaled analgesics are nitrous oxide and oxygen or trichlorethylene and air (trilene).

Local anesthetic

This is an injected anesthetic which numbs a specific area: **A perineal nerve block** is an injection into the stretched vaginal tissues to relieve pain as the baby's head presses

Acupuncture

This can help relieve pain and tension - it's thought by stimulating the release of endorphins (your body's own pain-killers), or by blocking the pain-messages passing through your nervous system. See an acupuncturist early in pregnancy if you want to use the technique during labour - not all are prepared to be available - and, if yours is to be a hospital birth, check with your doctor that your acupuncturist will be welcome.

Transcutaneous nerve stimulation (TNS) also works by blocking pain impulses to the brain - a small electric current is passed through electrodes on your back or abdomen. Some acupuncturists use TNS, and the equipment is found in some hospitals. Used right from the early stages of labour, it can be an effective form of pain relief and, if you can operate the equipment yourself, you can help control your own pain. It is safe and has no side-effects, though you'll be aware of a tingling sensation.

Massage

Low-back massage, correctly given, is relieving particularly towards the end of the first stage of labour. Try getting your partner to roll a tennis ball over your lumbar region

or use firm, circular movements over your lower back. This can be very helpful. Use stronger, firmer movements during contractions; sometimes just a hand placed on your lower back can make a difference. Light fingertip massage over your abdomen can be soothing. A little lavender or camomile oil can be rubbed onto your forehead, wrists and neck, or used for massage.

Herbalists
Raspberry leaf tea may be prescribed late in pregnancy as a herbal means of either toning up or relaxing the uterus but, as its effects vary from one woman to another, you should take expert advice rather than treating yourself. A herbalist may also suggest squaw vine (Mitchella repens)

Homoeopathy
Homoeopathic therapies might include caulophyllum, which comes from the same plant as squaw vine, to tone up the uterus beforehand, and arnica to ease any bruising that occurs during delivery. You can learn self-hypnosis techniques during pregnancy which you can apply in labour to help ease pain and tension.

down. The perineum may also be injected with a local anaesthetic before an episiotomy.

A pudendal nerve block removes feeling from the vulva and lower vagina and may be used when forceps are necessary.

These forms of analgesia would usually be available for both a hospital and a home confinement and may be used in conjunction with the methods of natural childbirth. Never feel you have 'failed' because you find you cannot take the pain - everyone has a different pain threshold and indeed, the pain you experience with one labour may be much greater than the pain of another. Natural childbirth has never pretended to be painless childbirth.

Epidural analgesia
An epidural removes rather than relieves the pain of labour without depriving you of full awareness and involvement. A local anaesthetic is injected into the lower spine to block the nerves that carry sensations of pain from the uterus to the brain.

While for many this is the perfect solution others may find it too clinical as well as limiting; with a catheter in your back and possibly a drip on your arm and a catheter in your bladder you certainly won't be having any sort of active birth! There may also be some loss of muscle power with feeling, leading to problems with pushing the baby out. However, if a forceps delivery is necessary, or even a Cesarean, an epidural already set up means this can be done without any further anesthetic. (An epidural can be a joy to those mothers destined always to have Cesareans who would otherwise never be conscious for the birth of their baby.)

Finding out
Whatever you decide on, make the most of whatever sources of support and information are available to you. Most hospitals run parentcraft classes covering exercises and relaxation techniques and demonstrations on breast-

feeding and baby bathing as well as arranging visits to the labour and delivery rooms so you can familiarize yourself with these. The National Childbirth Trust (NCT) also runs various ante-natal exercise and relaxation classes which are open to both you and your partner.

Involving your partner

Don't leave your partner out as the birth approaches. Some men feel hesitant about becoming fully involved in the birth although most now want to be present, but whether for purely emotional support or as an active supporter if you want to squat or stand in labour his contribution can be as significant now as it was earlier, at the conception.

On the other hand, if a man is really unhappy about doing breathing with you or even about being there in the labour room at all, be understanding. Equally, if you would really prefer him not to be there - you may feel happier with a close woman friend or your mother - discuss this with him. Both points of view are perfectly valid and should be respected.

Fetal heart monitoring

After week 20, the doctor or midwife will listen for the fetal heart at every ante-natal check-up to make sure that the baby is healthy and the heart rate normal. This is usually done with a fetal stethoscope or fetoscope, like an ear trumpet, pressed to your abdomen or sometimes with an electronic version. If an ultrasound apparatus known as sonicaid is available the fetal heart beat can be detected as early as ten weeks and this may be used in order to confirm pregnancy in some cases. The beauty of sonicaid to the expectant mother is that it amplifies the sound of the heart so that you can hear it clearly yourself.

The fetal heart beat is monitored throughout labour either using a fetoscope or by means of a belt fastened round your abdomen holding in place electrodes connected to an electronic fetal monitor (EFM). Sometimes an internal monitor, clipped to the baby's head is used (once the waters have broken and there is some dilation of the cervix) to record the heart beat while another is inserted between the baby and uterus wall to measure the contractions.

These machines are said to be more reliable than the human ear as far as picking up on fetal distress is concerned but this can lead to an increase in medical intervention in labour as well as severely limiting the mother's movements: even if you're on your back on a bed the electrodes keep slipping off so the monitor falters. Those in favour of these claim they reassure the mother that all is well.

Preparation exercises

While some people enjoy a relatively pain-free labour and delivery, the chances are that you'll experience pain of some sort at one stage or another. This may range from what you perceive as discomfort, to the kind that makes you feel as though you've had enough. Individuals differ in how they anticipate, experience and respond to pain - and external circumstances can make a difference, too. By preparing yourself mentally and physically for childbirth, you'll reduce your fear of the unknown and enhance your chances of making the whole experience a positive one. The earlier you start your preparations, the more confident you'll feel when the time comes.

Self-help

While you're pregnant, find out as much as you can about what you'll experience during childbirth. Nobody can tell you exactly how you're going to feel, but you can learn why your body's doing what it is (see pages 22-24) - and how you can help it. Once you know this, you can make sure that you're in the best possible physical condition to cope with childbirth and recover from it quickly. Regular physical exercise during pregnancy will tone up your muscles and help you handle stress and tension more effectively; simple relaxation techniques which you can apply during labour and delivery will also help.

Exercise

Regular aerobic exercise - walking, swimming, cycling - during pregnancy will help improve your circulation, strengthen your muscles, burn calories and increase your stamina. Your local sports or health centre may run regular classes especially for pregnant women, designed to tone your muscles and improve posture. Whatever exercise you do, don't do it on a full stomach - eat a light meal an hour or so before, or half-an-hour afterwards. Wear loose, comfortable clothing. Whether embarking on aerobic exercise or the daily ante-natal workout suggested overleaf, start off gently - and never strain. If anything hurts, stop.

Daily workout

While aerobic exercise will benefit your whole body, you'll be using muscles in childbirth you may not normally be aware of - and perhaps putting some additional strain on more familiar ones. By identifying, strengthening and toning them, you'll be able to release any tension they may be holding, increase their suppleness and help them work more efficiently. They'll also be in better shape to recover quickly from any stretching that occurs during labour and delivery.

You can do these exercises as a group in about 30 minutes but you can spread them out over the day if that's more convenient. Relax and breathe deeply for a few minutes before you start.

Head, neck and shoulders

If you're inclined to hold tension in the muscles of your face, neck and shoulders, you probably already know it. Identifying and getting rid of it aids relaxation at any time, and is especially important during childbirth when you can find yourself tensing up either between or during contractions.

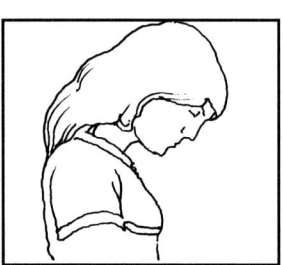

1. Kneel or sit comfortably on the floor, back straight. Don't hunch your shoulders. Let your head hang forwards and feel the nape of your neck relax.

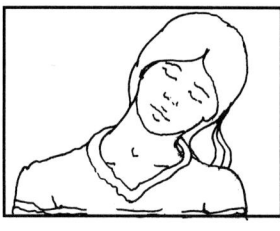

2. Breathing regularly and deeply, begin slowly to rotate your head and let its weight carry it round in a complete circle. Do this a couple of times, then repeat in the opposite direction. Don't jerk or strain for more movement than you can comfortably get - this will come with practice.

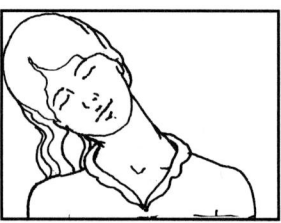

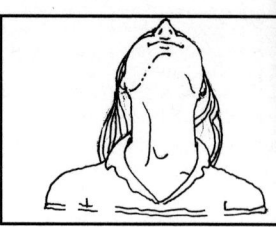

3. Slowly and gently allow your head to drop backwards. Release any tension in your jaws by opening your mouth wide for a few seconds. Bring your teeth together and feel the stretch in the front of your neck. Hold for a few seconds.

4. Keeping your shoulders facing forward, turn your head so that you're looking over your left shoulder - then repeat to the right.

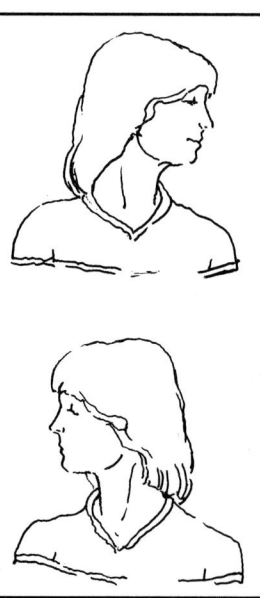

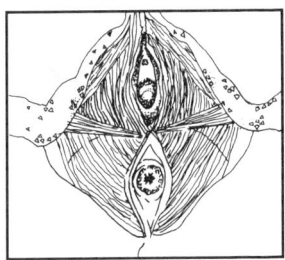

Pelvis, back and legs
Whatever position you choose for childbirth, you're going to need strength and flexibility here. Do these exercises as many times as you can, but stop if you feel strain rather than stretch.

Pelvic floor
The pelvic floor is the pear-shaped area of muscles between the pelvic bones around and inside the vagina (above) and are the muscles most under strain during pregnancy and birth. They include the muscles that control the entrance to the urethra and anus as well as the vagina and if they become weakened it can lead to urinary incontinence or prolapse of the uterus in later life. Too many women suffer from the former especially after they have had children so to strengthen these muscles before and restore them to their former springiness after the birth, first make sure you know which and where they are.

Lie on your back, tighten your buttock muscles, then pull up inside as if you're trying not to pass water - the muscles you feel tighten up are those of the pelvic floor. Repeat this exercise regularly, relaxing in between. You can also do it sitting or standing

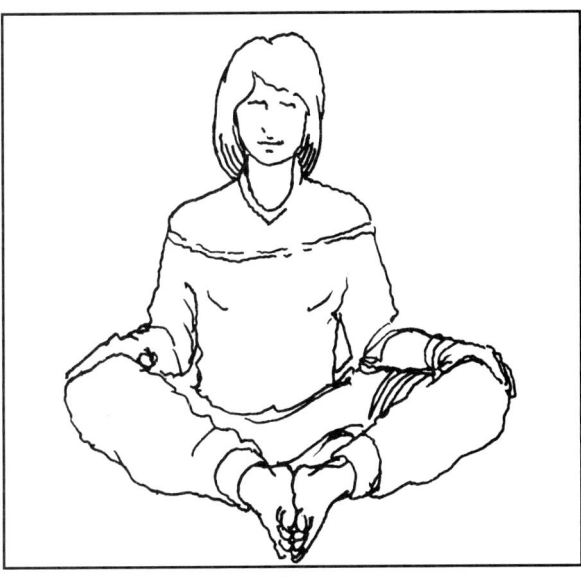

once you know what you're doing. A good way to test out the strength of your vaginal muscles in this area is actually to try and stop halfway through passing water. Also, try to contract the pelvic floor muscles gradually, as if they are drawing a lift up from the ground, floor by floor, then letting it down right again, floor by floor, until completely relaxed again.

1. Sit with your back straight, and your legs stretched out together in front. (Rest your lower back against a wall for extra support.) Bend your knees to bring your feet as near to your groin as you can (above), then turn your feet so that their soles are touching each other and the outsides are resting on the ground. Open out your thighs and lower your knees towards the

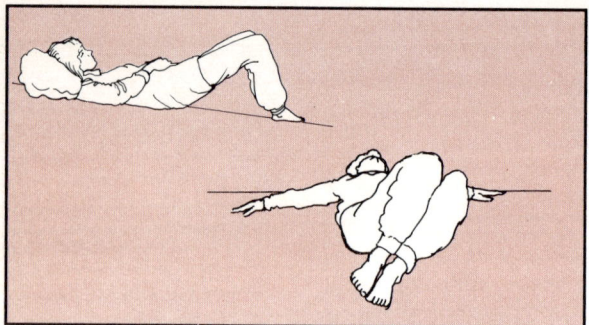

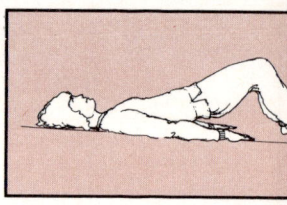

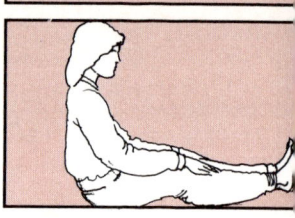

floor. Concentrate on breathing down towards the floor - relax the muscles in your legs and pelvic floor with each out-breath. Just before you inhale, stretch your spine upwards, but keep your shoulders relaxed. Hold the position for as long as it's comfortable: this will get easier as you become more supple.

2. Lie on your back, supporting your head and shoulders on a cushion or folded blanket. Bend your knees; keep your feet about 30 cm (12") apart, soles flat on the floor. Breathe out, press the small of your back into the floor; breathe in and relax. Repeat several times.

3. Still on your back, draw your knees up to your chest. Keep balanced by stretching your arms out to the side at right-angles to your body and pressing your palms to the floor. Keeping your knees together and your shoulders still, swing your knees to the left side, trying to touch the floor. Breathe out while you do this, then in as you return your knees to the centre. Repeat to the right; alternate several times.

4. Lie on your back, head and shoulders supported as before. Bend your knees; keep your feet about 30 cm (12") apart, soles flat on the floor. Keeping your shoulders flat, lift your body from your tailbone to your ribs off the floor, so that only your head, shoulders and feet are still in contact with it. Hold for five seconds, then gently lower your body to the floor - keeping your back as straight as you can. Remember to breathe slowly and easily throughout. Repeat several times.

5. Sit with your back supported against a wall. Point your toes, then flex your ankles so that your toes point at the ceiling. Repeat as often as you like - this is good for the circulation in your legs.

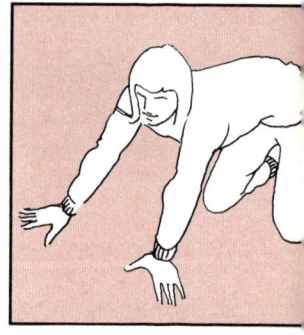

6. Turn over carefully, and bring yourself onto all fours. Put your hands shoulder-width apart; knees apart, too. Keep your back straight - don't let it sag - and your head and neck aligned with your spine. Breathe out, and hump your back by tightening your abdomen and buttocks so that you look like a camel, and allow your head to drop down. Gradually release your back and raise your head. Repeat several times. This is useful both during pregnancy and in

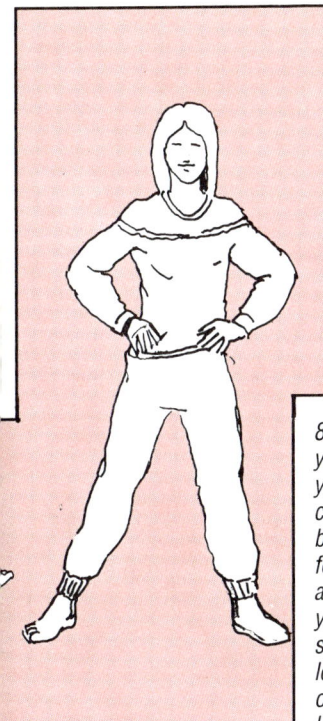

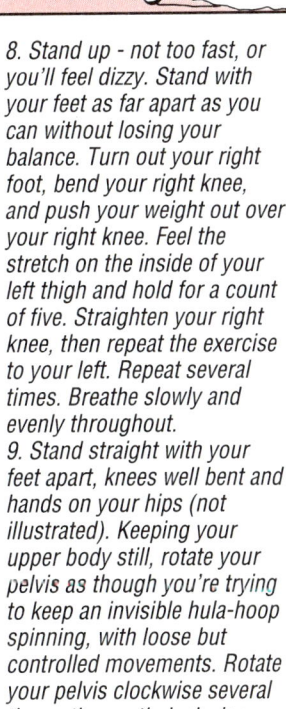

labour, as it relieves the pressure of your uterus on your back. Still on all fours, circle your bottom first to the left, then to the right, several times. Keep your back straight. Then push your hips to the left, feeling the stretch in your right side; repeat to the right and feel the stretch in your left side. Alternate several times, remembering to breathe regularly and keep your back straight.

8. Stand up - not too fast, or you'll feel dizzy. Stand with your feet as far apart as you can without losing your balance. Turn out your right foot, bend your right knee, and push your weight out over your right knee. Feel the stretch on the inside of your left thigh and hold for a count of five. Straighten your right knee, then repeat the exercise to your left. Repeat several times. Breathe slowly and evenly throughout.
9. Stand straight with your feet apart, knees well bent and hands on your hips (not illustrated). Keeping your upper body still, rotate your pelvis as though you're trying to keep an invisible hula-hoop spinning, with loose but controlled movements. Rotate your pelvis clockwise several times, then anti-clockwise.

10. Sit on the floor. (Rest your lower back against a wall if you find it hard to support your weight on your hands slightly behind you.) Keeping your legs straight, stretch them as far apart as you can. Point your toes, then flex your ankles so that your toes point at the ceiling. Repeat as often as you like - this is good for the circulation in your legs, and improves suppleness in your inner thighs.
11. Finish off gently by repeating the 'head, neck and shoulders' exercise; sit comfortably for a few minutes, breathing deeply and regularly.

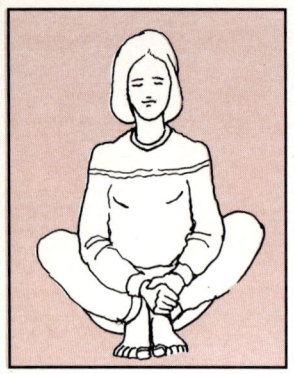

Squatting

You may also want to get used to squatting in preparation for the birth. Begin by lowering yourself onto a couple of cushions with your back against a wall for support. Squatting steadily with heels flat on the ground may take a while to achieve. When you can do this remember to keep your back straight and press out with your elbows against your inner thighs.

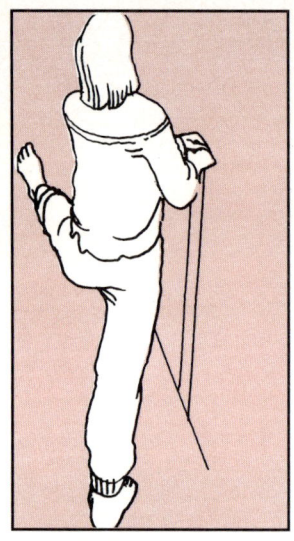

Hips and abdomen

Stand holding on to something steady and raise one leg as high as you can without it being a strain. Then swing it back and forth, remembering to keep both legs straight as you do so. Repeat with other leg.

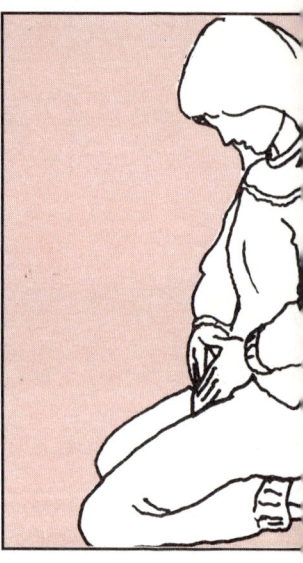

1. Find somewhere quiet and well ventilated - outdoors, if it's warm enough. It's best not to eat for an hour beforehand. Experiment until you find a comfortable position - kneeling with your bottom on your heels and knees slightly apart, sitting cross-legged on the floor against a wall, or upright on a straight-backed chair with your feet flat on the floor. Whatever position you choose, ensure you can keep your back straight without straining, then let your chin

Breathing for relaxation

It's worth learning how to relax - physically and mentally - during pregnancy, so that you can use relaxation and controlled breathing techniques to help cope with any stress or pain you may experience during childbirth.

Practise every day; use this kind of controlled breathing while you're doing your exercise workout, and whenever you find yourself getting tense.

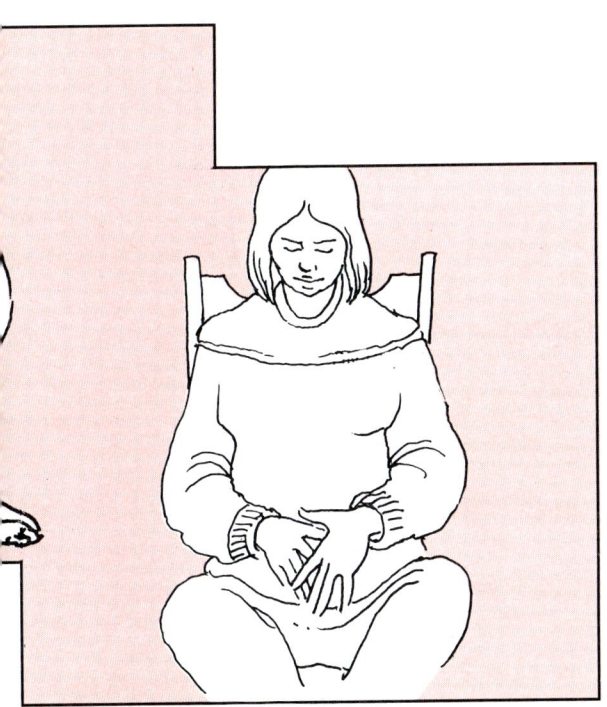

Breathing for labour
First stage
Relax in a comfortable position and focus attention on your breathing. As a contraction begins, concentrate on exhaling through your mouth and releasing tension. Imagine your body opening; feel your pelvic floor muscles relax. At the end of each out-breath, remain empty for a few moments and allow the in-breath to begin. Repeat through each contraction.

Second stage
You won't know what's best for you until you feel the urge to push. Then you can either take a deep breath, hold it and push as long as you can - or relax, breathe deeply and let your body do the work. Again, it helps to imagine your body opening and 'feel' your baby waiting to be born.

drop gently towards your chest.
2. Place your hands gently on your lower abdomen, and become aware of the rhythm of your breathing. Feel your belly move away from your hands with each out-breath.
3. Breathe out slowly through your mouth; empty your lungs. Rest like this for a few
moments. When you're ready, breathe in gently through your nose - again, into your belly rather than your chest - and feel your belly expand towards your hands.
4. Continue to breathe like this, one breath flowing into the next. As you get used to it, you'll find it brings a sense of calmness.

Post-natal

After the birth you will also want to exercise the abdominal muscles then those of the lower back and thighs. It is also important to continue to do the pelvic floor exercises described on page 51. Keep tensing and relaxing the pelvic floor throughout the day, at any time, anywhere. Nobody will know that you are doing it (unless you are pulling a face, or making love at the time). You can do the exercises within days of delivery. Set time aside to do them for five minutes a session first thing in the morning, in the middle of the day and at some time in the evening. Use the relaxation techniques you learnt in ante-natal class to unwind at the end of your exercise session. (If you have had a Cesarian section, the physiotherapist at the hospital will advise you on when you can begin working on the abdominal muscles.)

It will probably take you a full three months to get back into shape after having a baby, perhaps a little longer. If you find that after this time you are still not back to the weight you were before pregnancy, you can start thinking about cutting down on your calorie intake.

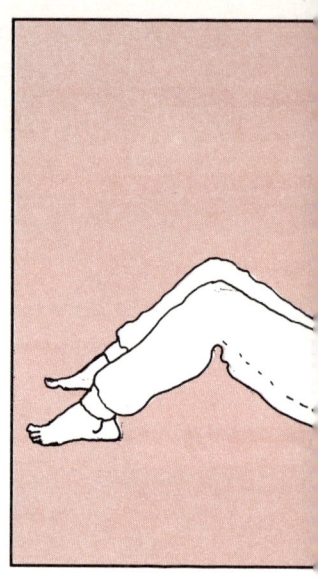

Abdomen (left)

Lie on your back and pull in your abdominal muscles. Slide the heel of one leg away from you then pull the whole leg in towards you. Repeat with other leg.

Lie with knee bent and feet flat. Pull in your abdominal muscles then reach as far as you can with one hand across the other side of the your body. Repeat with other hand.

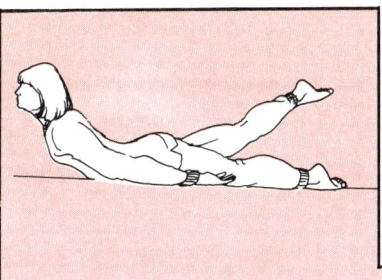

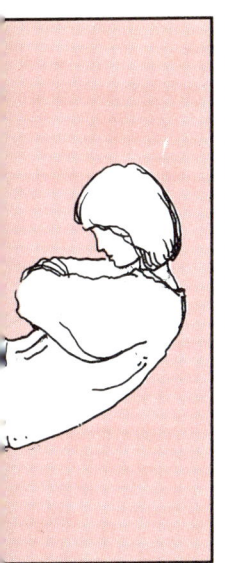

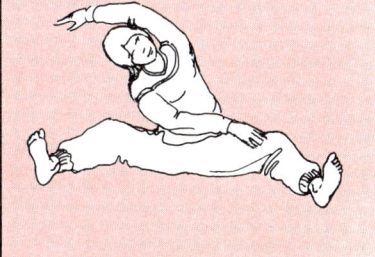

Abdomen (above)
Sit with your feet on the floor, knees bent, and heels parallel about hip distance apart. Cross your arms in front of you and slowly curl down to a lying position. Feel the pull in your stomach muscles.
It is important that your back slowly uncurls in contact with the floor so that you do not strain it.

Place your hands onto your thighs and slowly slide them towards your knees as you pull up into a sitting position. Again, recurl your back slowly.

Lower back and thighs (top and above)
Lie face down with arms by your sides then raise your head and one leg (straight) up off the ground. Hold then relax. Repeat with other leg. Sit with your legs as wide open as possible and feet flexed (toes pointing upwards). Keeping your back absolutely straight, lift one arm over your head and bend as far sideways as you can without straining yourself; don't let your hips rise up off the ground. Repeat with the other arm.

Common problems

Adding extra foods rich in iron, folic acid and vitamin B_{12} to your daily diet helps reduce the risk of anemia:

• Iron
Cherry juice; seaweeds; brewer's yeast powder; brown meats - including liver, black pudding, kidney; green leafy vegetables; whole grains - e.g. in wholemeal bread and breakfast cereals; pulses; sprouted seeds and grains; sunflower seeds; dried fruits; watermelon; egg yolk; nuts; mushrooms; beetroot; molasses.

• Folic acid
Dark leafy greens; brewer's yeast and yeast extract; root vegetables; whole grains and wheatgerm; peanuts and almonds; oysters; salmon; whole milk; dates; mushrooms; tomato puree; orange juice; liver. Folic acid tends to be lost in cooking: retain it by adding cooking-liquids to soups or stock.

• Vitamin B_{12}
Brewer's yeast and yeast extracts; dairy produce; fish; offal; seaweeds; wheatgerm; oysters; beef; pork.

Use fresh culinary herbs like watercress, chives, lovage and fennel in a daily salad and sprinkle it with parsley (don't

A number of common problems beset even the most normal pregnancies, but most can be combated with simple self-help approaches. A number of people find that complementary and alternative therapies offer relief for many of these problems, and suggestions for this type of approach are given in the tinted columns of this section.

Anemia

If you are always tired and lacking in energy as well as perhaps looking rather pale, you may well be anemic. This means that your blood hemoglobin level is low and this is tested when you book in for antenatal care and later, at about 30 then 36 weeks (a level below 10 g is not now acceptable).

Hemoglobin performs a vital function carrying oxygen round the body, and to the growing baby, and is contained in the red blood cells.

During pregnancy anemia can result from the increase in the volume of blood in your body and the dilution of red blood cell concentration with extra plasma (fluid). Sometimes, however, there is an overall increase in red blood cells, especially if you are eating properly.

A second reason for anemia in pregnancy is that an essential ingredient of hemoglobin is iron, which the growing fetus is taking for itself - one-third of a pregnant woman's iron reserves passes over to her baby. If you are anemic, to boost your hemoglobin level and to ensure both your baby and you have enough iron you will be given supplements of iron and folic acid, which also aids the manufacture of new blood cells.

These supplements are sometimes prescribed routinely though a healthy and well-nourished woman may have sufficient iron reserves in her body to cope with the extra demands of pregnancy.

Many women, however, do enter pregnancy with no iron reserves, especially if they have heavy periods. The only drawback of iron pills is that they often give rise to heartburn and constipation though change to a different type of iron pill will sometimes solve the problem. You may be offered iron injections as an alternative if your level is particularly low or fails to rise after a spell on iron.

To avoid anemia, eat a well-balanced diet including plenty of foods rich in iron; these include red meat, kidney and liver, shellfish, green leafy vegetables, mushrooms and beetroot, whole foods such as grains and pulses, sprouted seeds and grains, dried fruit, nuts, egg yolks and molasses. You might also consider avoiding drinking tea with or soon after a meal as this may inhibit the absorption or iron from that meal.

Anxiety

Pregnancy is not only a time for joyous anticipation. You may be outwardly blooming while inwardly full of anxiety; few women get through their nine months without some niggling worry which may seem foolish to someone else but is real nonetheless.

You are committed to having a baby and may worry that you have made a mistake: will it ruin your relationship with your partner; will he, can he still love you when you're big and ungainly? - and what about your job, your independence?

You may also worry about coping when the new baby arrives: will you be able to feed and care for him or her properly - what if you make some dreadful mistake? And if you have other children, how will they react and will you find space in your heart to love the new baby as much as you do them?

But among the most common anxieties to beset the expectant mother are those connected with labour, especially with losing control and coping with pains: will you make a scene, screaming? - what if the pain becomes too great too bear? - what if I empty my bowels in front of everyone? - what if I just can't do it?

Finally there can be very few mothers who have not at some point been anxious about their baby being born with some abnormality, however small. Pregnancy is a period of transition and both your body and mind are preparing for the new baby; it is only natural that you should think - and worry - about what the future holds. But try not to let your anxiety get out of hand and don't

use too much, as it's sometimes used in large quantities to cause abortion); elderberries can be stewed with apples and blackberries. Absorption of iron can be helped by eating foods rich in vitamin C at the same meal - a salad with an omelette, for example, or following an egg sandwich by an orange. It's hindered by coffee, strong tea and cola so avoid drinking these with or after meals. If you're vegetarian, or find that high doses of iron in the form of supplements cause heartburn and constipation, try an organic iron tonic (available from health-food stores). Some homoeopathic treatments may improve your body's ability to absorb iron.

Backache

Any 'alternative' practitioner will want to identify the reasons for pain before treating it. Consulting an osteopath or chiropractor immediately if you experience sudden, acute pain may well mean that you stop it becoming chronic. You'll also get advice on remedial exercises and any changes to your posture or working positions that will help. Good results are often achieved when manipulative therapy is combined with relaxation techniques. The Alexander Technique can help improve your posture, and so prevent problems.

Acupuncture and hypnotherapy can help relieve pain, so may acupressure (ask an acupuncturist or masseur for advice). Naturopathic hydrotherapy for aching or stiffness might take the form of hot and cold fomentations (moist compresses, usually a towel wrung out in water) - a hot one applied to the site of the pain for three minutes followed by a cold one for one minute, repeated over 20-30 minutes at least once a day. This kind of stiffness can improve with gentle exercise, but stop if it hurts.

If your backache is the result of tension rather than any structural problem, both acupressure and massage can be soothing and relaxing.

suppress it: speak up, tell your partner and the doctor or midwife you see for ante-natal care about your fears. They may not be able to give iron-clad reassurances but they may offer information or words of experience that help. Find out as much as you can about childbirth and child care from other mothers and from books - fear is often a result of ignorance - but don't frighten yourself listening to old wives' tales or look for one-in-a million horror cases in obstetric textbooks! Accept that your anxiety is normal and just try to be positive: things usually work out all right and even when they don't people usually cope.

Backache

The hormone progesterone produced by the placenta serves to soften and stretch the ligaments of the body so that in labour the pelvic joints will be able to move freely to let the baby through. In the process the ligaments of the spine are also affected with the result that it becomes easier to overstrain the lower joints, especially those between spine and pelvis.

Pregnant women tend to throw back their shoulders to offset the load they carry in front which puts great strain on the lower back and frequently results in discomfort, sometimes quite acute. To prevent backache, try to stand upright, holding in as far as possible both buttocks and abdomen, and when sitting don't slouch with your back unsupported, try to keep your back straight. You would be well-advised to avoid wearing high-heeled shoes as these throw your whole body forward, putting even more strain on the spinal muscles, and sleep if possible on a firm mattress.

In the later months try to avoid standing or bending over for any length of time, or carrying heavy shopping bags, and get plenty of rest. Last, keep an eye on your weight: excessive weight gain will surely lead to bad posture and thus backache.

If you have a history of back problems see your doctor about any backache. Mention it in any case at your ante-natal visit.

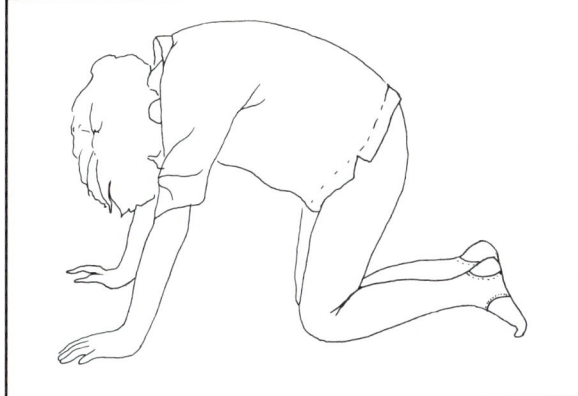

To relieve backache, get down onto all fours and arch your back gently upwards.

Breathlessness

Occasional breathlessness after some exertion is not un-common at any stage of pregnancy but becomes generally more marked and more frequent in a greater number of women in the last ten weeks. This is because the enlarging uterus forces the diaphragm up into the chest so that there is simply less room for you to breathe efficiently. There is no need to worry about it.

If however you find yourself short of breath when you haven't really exerted yourself it may be that you are simply unfit but another possible cause is anemia so see your doctor about it. You should certainly seek his advice if your breathlessness comes on suddenly or is associated with any sort of bad cough, cold or fever.

If you think you are unfit (and have ruled out other possibilities) try to get a bit more exercise on a regular basis - for instance gentle walking or swimming - but don't overdo it or you will end up with a different set of problems! If you are short of breath at night prop yourself up in bed with a couple of pillows to reduce the pressure of the uterus on your diaphragm. If you are having your first baby you may notice some relief at about thirty-six

Breathlessness
Treatment for breathlessness depends on whether the cause is physical or psychological. If you react to anxiety or stress by breathing fast and less deeply than usual, you may end up feeling that you can't get enough air - and panicky. The result can be dizziness, chest pain or additional symptoms of stress.

Acupuncture treatment depends on causes, and you might find that acupressure - to the point in the hollow between the tendons of your thumb that is visible when you spread your hand wide - is helpful. Hypnotherapy would try to identify any underlying causes of anxiety, and could also be used to help you modify your breathing patterns in times of stress. During hypnotherapy you could well be taught a variation of the self-help relaxation technique described in the main text overleaf. Tea made by adding a cupful of boiling water to 5-10 ml (1-2 teaspoons) of chopped limeblossom or lemon balm will help you relax. The relaxing effects of the postural re-education which is part of the Alexander Technique may be beneficial.

If your breathlessness is a result of catarrhal congestion, naturopathy suggests you should cut down your intake of dairy produce and base

your diet on plenty of fruit, vegetables and whole grains. Hot and cold fomentations (see Backache) may help, and you can increase the capacity of your lungs by taking regular exercise such as walking or swimming.

Constipation

The connection between constipation and lack of dietary fibre is now well established. Increasing your intake of fibre by eating unpeeled (washed) fresh fruit and steamed or raw vegetables helps; other fibre-rich foods include wholemeal bread and wholegrain breakfast cereals. Increasing your fluid intake to two litres a day is a simple preventative measure.

Sprinkling bran on refined carbohydrates makes less sense than eating more food in its natural state: naturopaths say that bran can be used as an emergency measure - along with other natural laxatives like dried fruits or linseed - but suggest that long-term use in pregnancy isn't a good idea as it can lock essential minerals into compounds your body can't absorb. The occasional bout of constipation can be relieved by eating prunes or dried fruit.

Acupuncturists don't prescribe laxatives, but work to restore correct energy

weeks as the baby's head descends into the pelvis ('engages'), giving the diaphragm a chance to descend a little again.

To relax, choose a time and place when you know you won't be disturbed. Make it somewhere quiet - at least while you're getting the hang of this. Later you'll even be able to use this technique when conditions aren't ideal. Loosen any tight clothing; sit or lie down comfortably. Concentrate on tightening each muscle in turn, working methodically from your toes to your head. This way you'll become conscious of any physical tension you're holding. Loosen each muscle, and feel your body become heavy.

Stay like this for 10 or 15 minutes, feeling yourself breathing slowly and calmly. Try and keep your mind empty of unwelcome thoughts - either by concentrating on your breathing or an image that reminds you of something pleasant, or simply by chasing them out when they do occur.

Constipation

A tendency to constipation is often noticed in pregnancy and the main reason is, again, the relaxing action of the hormone progesterone on body muscle. This time it is the smooth (involuntary) muscle of the intestine that is affected, reducing its ability to propel its contents along towards the rectum and anus (back passage). In later pregnancy, pressure on the lower bowel from the enlarged uterus contributes to the problem.

It is only a tendency, however, and if you are eating plenty of roughage you are unlikely to become constipated. This means eating brown bread and rice instead of white, fresh fruit (unpeeled), vegetables and salads. The bulk fibrous foods provide stimulates the lower bowel into working and expelling its contents. Also drink plenty of fluids, especially tap water or mineral water.

The iron pills given ante-natally often cause constipation; ask for a different type if yours do. Don't start taking laxatives; they do as much harm as good as well as, very occasionally, provoking miscarriage where a very strong dose has been taken.

Cramp

Cramp is caused by prolonged tightening of a group of muscles and can be very painful. In pregnancy it is most common in the thigh, calf and foot, especially in the last ten weeks and especially at night when you may wake up crying out with the pain.

No one knows what causes cramp though there is thought to be a link with a low level of calcium or salt in the blood. If you persistently suffer from cramp your doctor may suggest increasing your intake of either or both of these substances. Don't increase your salt consumption, however, without his advice; too much salt is not good for pregnant women. Daytime leg cramps may be associated with varicose veins; consult your doctor.

To deal with cramp when it happens, firmly massage the affected muscles straight away and flex the foot

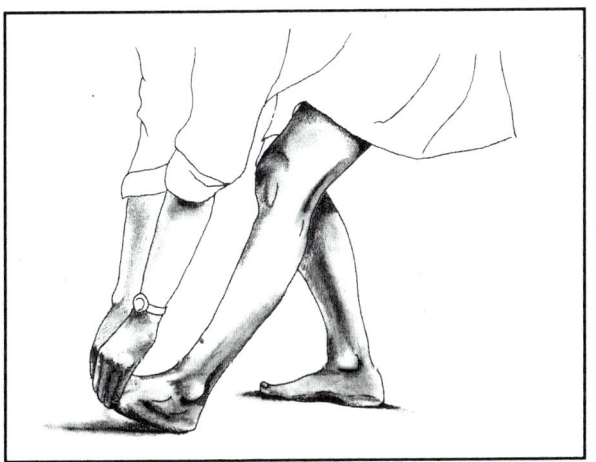

For the occasional acute attack, stretching the muscle against the contraction will help - but you probably won't enjoy it much to begin with.

balances in the digestive organs. They can also suggest balanced diets to deal with specific types of constipation, and show you how to apply effective acupressure. Gentle massage starting at the bottom right-hand side of your abdomen, across your diaphragm and down the left side of your abdomen may stimulate your colon - but don't use heavy pressure.

A herbal practitioner may suggest temporary remedies in the form of natural laxatives - adding soaked linseed to breakfast cereal, taking senna pods, or drinking an infusion of dandelion leaves and roots - but take expert advice before treating yourself. Different remedies are prescribed for different kinds of constipation. A homoeopath may suggest nux vomica.

Help yourself by always going to the toilet when your body says you should, and avoid straining. Make sure you're getting enough exercise, especially for your abdominal muscles.

Cramp
In hot weather, increase your intake of salt and calcium-rich foods such as whole milk and milk products, dark green leafy vegetables, shellfish, salmon, black treacle, prunes, nuts, egg yolk, sprouted seeds and grains, oranges, papayas, watermelon and carrots. Avoid

wearing high-heeled shoes, and - if night-time cramps are a problem - try sleeping on a firmer surface.

Massage can encourage the circulation of blood to the affected area; hot and cold fomentations (see Backache) will have a similar effect. A herbalist may suggest taking regular doses of Viburnum opulus (cramp bark), or giving yourself mustard footbaths three times a week. To do this, dissolve 15 ml (1 tablespoon) mustard powder into a bowl containing enough water to cover your feet. Bathe them for three minutes, splashing the water over your calves as well.

Homoeopathic remedies vary according to the kind of symptoms you have: arnica when your cramp is part of general tiredness; calcarea carbonica when it's associated with damp, cold feet and a tendency to be overweight; nux vomica for night-time cramps with no apparent cause. Consult a homoeopath rather than treating yourself.

Faintness
Regularly contract and relax the muscles of your buttocks to get your blood flowing to your brain, and try lying on your side instead of your back when you're in bed so that the weight of your uterus doesn't press on the large blood vessels.

(bend it up towards you). This should relieve the pain quite quickly though a dull ache may remain for some time. (Get someone to do this for you if you can; it's not easy doing it yourself when you are pregnant).

Fainting

A degree of relaxation of the muscle in the heart and blood vessels (caused by progesterone released by the placenta) sometimes results in a drop in your blood pressure - the blood isn't being pumped round so efficiently - and this may lead to fainting. This is especially likely to happen if you have been standing for some time so that the blood has gathered in your legs, starving the brain. The growing uterus is also making great demands on your blood supply at this time, contributing to the reduction in blood pressure.

But fainting is more than just a result of this lack of supply, it is a response to it: when you fall your head is brought down level with your heart and the head's blood supply is automatically restored. Don't worry if this happens to you; it is very common in early pregnancy although many women find they only feel faint. In fact low blood pressure is generally a good thing in pregnancy. The only possible danger is of hurting yourself if you fall, so if you do feel lightheaded, sit down quickly and take a few deep breaths. Avoid standing for long periods, for instance in queues.

This sort of faintness or dizziness may also come over you when you stand after sitting for some time or getting up from bed (lying on your side is better than on your back if you suffer from faintness as this avoids the uterus pressing down on the large blood vessels in your back). Some women continue to feel the effects of low blood pressure throughout their pregnancy though the blood pressure usually returns to normal after about fourteen weeks as the volume of blood circulating round the body increases to cope. Blood pressure will be tested at every ante-natal visit and if you feel faint persistently make a point of mentioning it to the doctor or midwife. Avoiding extreme heat and alcohol can help but, if you do feel faint, sit down quickly so you don't fall and hurt yourself.

Fatigue and tiredness

In the first months especially it is not uncommon for a normally energetic woman to feel permanently tired and lethargic, uninterested even in what is going on around her, and such fatigue is usually seen as 'nature's way' of making her slow down. She is probably experiencing a sudden drop in blood pressure (see Fainting), her heart is having to work much harder and hormonal changes may affect her energy level too. Anemia is another possible cause of tiredness in pregnancy, as are nausea and heart-burn which affect how much nourishment she is getting.

The greatest lassitude is usually felt between six and fourteen weeks, though in second or later pregnancies it lasts longer and is more severe - up to twenty weeks in some cases. All you can do is get plenty of rest, not only by sleeping but by taking it easy and resting with your feet up in the afternoon, indeed whenever and wherever you can. Don't try to fight your fatigue; you will only make yourself miserable and probably those around you too.

Many mothers-to-be find that they regain energy and feel on top of the world during the middle section of their pregnancy. Take care though not to exhaust yourself. As you increase in size and weight fatigue usually catches up towards the end of term; again, don't force yourself to do more than you feel is enough, however much or little that is.

Gum disorders

Because of the progesterone in the body during pregnancy the gums often soften and become almost spongy. In this state they are vulnerable, easily damaged by harsh brushing, for instance, and are prone to infection. They may become red and swollen and recede from the base of the teeth, exposing them to decay.

For this reason it is important to maintain a high level of dental hygiene in pregnancy; brushing with a soft

Fatigue
Chronic fatigue in pregnancy may simply be a side-effect of not being able to get comfortable enough to sleep properly. If other causes exist - like stress or anxiety - a holistic approach can identify them and suggest remedies.

The Alexander Technique can be useful when fatigue is the result of poor posture; hypnotherapy and massage are helpful in dealing with tiredness caused by stress.

If fatigue is caused by poor sleep-quality, aromatherapy suggests that sprinkling a few drops of oil of lavender, camomile or marjoram in your bath will help you relax - or you can drop some on your pillow. Herbal remedies might include peppermint tea two or three times a day, said to be relaxing. There are a number of homoeopathic remedies for insomnia, but they depend on the reasons for it - consult an expert to find out which would be best for you.

Because anemia can be a cause of chronic fatigue, it's important to seek professional help. In this case, a naturopath might suggest dietary adjustments - like restricted intake of sugar and refined carbohydrates, and an increase of protein from whole grains and pulses.

Gum disorders
Naturopathic theory suggests

that you should follow a low-sugar diet, avoid sugary and sticky foods between meals, and eat plenty of chewy foods to encourage the production of saliva which protects your mouth from harmful bacteria. You can make a two-stage mouthwash by adding 10 ml (2 teaspoons) 20-vol hydrogen peroxide to 120 ml (4 fl oz) hot water. Use all this mixture, squeezing it between your teeth, then spit it out - don't swallow it. Then add 5 ml (1 teaspoon) Milton fluid to another 120 ml hot water, and rinse your mouth out several times. Again, don't swallow this mixture, and don't rinse out with anything else afterwards.

You can make a herbal mouthwash with 5-10 ml (1-2 teaspoons) of a mixture of thyme and sage to a cup of hot water - again, rinse but don't swallow, as sage can have an adverse effect on the production of breast milk.

Headaches

Any 'alternative' practitioner will concentrate first on identifying their cause rather than simply suppressing the pain. Once the reason for the headaches is clear, treatment can begin.

By correcting any postural problems, the Alexander Technique can help prevent the headaches that arise as a

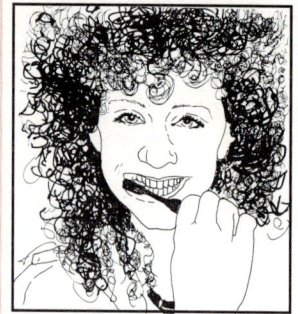

Use dental floss regularly. Work it down gently between the gum margin and the tooth, then slide it up the edge of the tooth before working back down the other side. If the floss becomes blood-stained, it means that you have an area of gingivitis and you need to pay particular attention to this part of your mouth.

During pregnancy the gums tend to be slightly more puffy. This means that you must be even more rigorous about oral hygiene. Loosen the plaque from the gum edge with small, circular movements before flicking the brush downwards away from the gums.

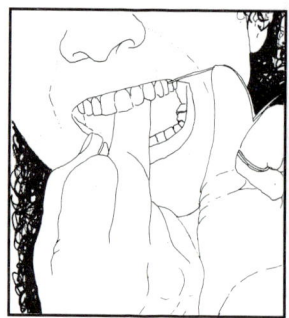

nylon brush, gently using dental floss between the teeth, and perhaps also rinsing out with a mouthwash of one part hydrogen peroxide to five parts water. Visit the dentist (dental care is free while you're pregnant), but make sure that if you need an X-ray you are protected below the neck by a screen or lead apron.

Eat foods rich in calcium to strengthen the teeth - milk and its derivatives being the most obvious - and avoid sweet things, especially between meals. Eat fresh fruit and vegetables for vitamins; apples will also help to harden your gums.

Headaches

Headaches can be the result of tension, anxiety or stress as well as physical problems caused by eye strain or poor posture. A number of women find that they suffer more from headaches during pregnancy, but are anxious about taking the ordinary across-the-counter remedies, particularly during the first three months of pregnancy.

If you are troubled continually by headaches, or, if you suffer from migraines, find that your pattern of migraine has altered, consult your doctor who will be able to advise you on the safest type of painkiller to take.

Planning ahead can help you avoid unnecessary tension, rush and anxiety, and regular relaxation exercises can also help (see Breathlessness for an example).

Heartburn

Progesterone relaxes the valve at the upper end of the stomach so that the stomach contents, which are normally acid, escape up into the lower part of the oesophagus (food pipe or gullet), irritating its sensitive lining. The lining becomes inflamed so that the next escape of gastric acid results in the burning sensation we call heartburn. It is not strictly indigestion although the medicines used are similar.

The enlarging uterus contributes to the problem by putting upward pressure on the stomach, and by pushing out the lower ribs so that the gap in the diaphragm through which the oesophagus passes is opened slightly making it easier for the acid to escape up the gullet. This is why heartburn occurs or worsens as you gain in bulk - and why you are more likely to suffer from it if you are carrying twins or just excess weight

The answer is not to dose yourself up with strong antacids as the stomach will react to their alkali by becoming even more acid. Instead, take a small dose, then suck an antacid: put half a tablet between cheek and gum and just let it dissolve slowly over a couple of hours. This should give the inflammation a chance to subside. Ask your doctor what alkali to take; milk of magnesia is usually acceptable.

Also, don't overload your stomach - take small meals more often - and avoid spicy or fried foods, and possibly also alcohol. Try sipping milk, or eat yogurt, to

result of muscular tension, while osteopathy and chiropractic can use massage, mobilization of stiff joints and manipulation to relieve the 'tension-muscular contraction-headache-increased tension' cycle. Swedish or Shiatsu massage can ease tension and promote relaxation. Practitioners can also suggest helpful changes to posture or habitual working positions.

To the acupuncturist, the precise site of headaches can indicate the meridians where some imbalance is present. You may get temporary relief in acute cases by applying acupressure to points at the base of your skull, to your forehead for frontal headaches, and to your temples. Ask an acupuncturist or masseur to show you how.

Herbal treatment also depends on the cause of your headaches, and their specific symptoms. Infusions - made by adding 0.5 litres (1 pint) boiling water to 25 g (1 oz) freshly-chopped leaves or flowers of the herb, then straining before drinking - of limeblossom or lavender may be suggested for headaches resulting from stress or nervous tension. A drop of lavender oil massaged gently into your temples is soothing.

Peppermint tea is useful, and the leaves of the herb can be used in a poultice and applied to the site of the pain. Make one by crushing about 60 g (2 oz) of the leaves and mixing them into a spreadable paste with a little hot water; add some flour, cornmeal or bran if necessary to make it go further. Sandwich the paste in a thin cloth before applying it to your skin. Rue, used in a compress or as an eyebath, can ease headaches caused by eyestrain. A medical herbalist can advise on what's best for you. Homoeopathic remedies are also specific to you as an individual.

Hydrotherapy can help relieve muscular tension - try applying hot and cold fomentations (see Backache) to your neck and shoulders, or cold compresses to your forehead. Naturopaths also suggest that headache-sufferers, who tend to be competitive, highly-motivated people, can benefit from trying to take a more relaxed approach to life.

Heartburn, indigestion and flatulence
Try modifying your lifestyle if it tends to be rushed and stressful. Avoid alcohol and highly-spiced or fried foods, and eat little and often. Chew your food well, and avoid drinking with your meals. Don't let tight clothing put pressure on your abdomen. If heartburn tends to strike at

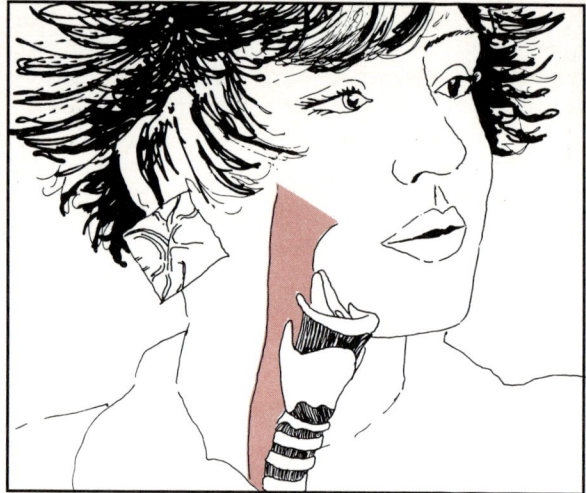

Heartburn occurs when stomach acid irritates the lining of the oesophagus. It happens more frequently in late pregnancy because of the increased abdominal pressure.

neutralize the acid.

Don't eat immediately before bedtime and in bed prop yourself up on several pillows to keep your head above your chest. In the day try to maintain a good upright posture and avoid bending over if possible - this often triggers off heartburn.

Hemorrhoids (piles)

Hemorrhoids are distended veins in and around the anus. They are usually caused by excessive straining to empty the bowel due to constipation and exacerbated in pregnancy by the pressure of the enlarging uterus and later of the baby's head in the pelvis, restricting the flow of blood back from this area. Progesterone relaxes the blood vessel muscle, as it does all body muscle in pregnancy, which encourages dilatation of the veins.

Hemorrhoids can also arise from, or worsen, with the strain put on the veins during the second stage of labour. They usually settle down afterwards but will become worse with each successive pregnancy, sometimes becoming permanent. Signs of hemorrhoids are soreness and a lump in the anus with pain and bleeding when you empty your bowels.

If the piles become really painful your doctor may prescribe an ointment or suppositories to help but the basic treatment really is up to you - preventing constipation (see above). Should the hemorrhoids protrude from the anus push them back in gently with your finger. If they are really painful apply an ice-pack and use a rubber-ring as a cushion to sit on.

A sensible diet which provides enough dietary fibre will help prevent piles, or ease discomfort if they do occur. High-fibre foods (see Constipation) and plenty of fluids will help keep stools soft and easy to pass. It's important to try and avoid straining when defecating - try to keep relaxed. You may find that deep breathing helps, and that regular pelvic floor exercises improve muscle tone and control.

Insomnia

Just when you need all the sleep you can get, insomnia can set in. You may not be able to get to sleep in the first place because you can't get comfortable or have heartburn, or you may be unable to doze off again having been woken by the baby kicking or the need to go to the toilet.

Aim to go to bed already relaxed - by a soak in the bath or a hot milky drink - and then practise your relaxation technique once in bed. Don't rush around up to the last minute then lie in bed making lists of things you've got to do and expect your mind to be able to turn off the instant you shut your eyes.

Adapt your usual sleeping position to suit your shape - lying on the back is generally uncomfortable and restricts the blood flow while lying on your front isn't possible after a certain point. Lie on your side with a pillow beneath your abdomen to support it and perhaps another between your knees and thighs. Sleeping propped up against a bank of pillows is especially comfortable if you suffer from heartburn. If persistent backache is your prob-

night, try having a milky drink before you go to bed and lying propped up instead of flat. Acupuncture can investigate the general efficiency of your digestive system before treating specific imbalances. Many culinary herbs and spices are known to aid digestion: use caraway and fennel seeds, marjoram and thyme in your cooking, and try chewing (but not swallowing) coriander seeds before and after meals. Peppermint tea is helpful, so is aniseed. You can make a tea with 5-10 ml (1-2 teaspoons) of chopped meadowsweet to 0.5 litres (1 pint) boiling water, and sip it on and off during the day. Homoeopathic remedies take all your symptoms into account and vary from one individual to another, so expert advice is essential. Consult a naturopath for dietary advice; hot and cold fomentations can help relieve pain or colic.

Hemorrhoids (piles)
Herbal treatment for piles might include pilewort (lesser celandine) ointment which relieves pain, eases inflammation and reduces the piles. You can apply this two or three times a day, and after each bowel movement. Distilled witch hazel may reduce discomfort. Homoeopathic remedies are available in the form of

ointments or suppositories: consult a practitioner for advice.

Naturopaths suggest that hydrotherapy can help ease discomfort. Try bathing the affected area alternately with hot and cold water, sitting in a cold hip-bath, sponging with ice-cold water or applying ice-packs.

Nausea and sickness
Try to get plenty of rest during the day, and one or two early nights a week. Eat small, regular meals and avoid highly-spiced or fatty foods. Go for soups and other liquid food if you find it hard to keep anything down, and drink water and fruit juice rather than tea and coffee. You may find that deep breathing helps diminish feelings of nausea, and peppermint tea is very soothing.

Though some traditional acupuncturists prefer not to treat nausea and vomiting during pregnancy, acupuncture can be useful in cases of severe vomiting - but usually only temporarily. If your sickness is the result of being under stress, hypnotherapy may help; simple relaxation exercises will relieve tension.

lem get a new firm mattress or put planks beneath your present one to firm it up.

To avoid being woken by the need to go to the toilet cut down on your fluid intake in the last couple of hours before bed; it may be worth it. There's not much you can do about the baby's movements; if these are the cause of your awakening, accept it. Sit up and read a book, listen to the radio or cassette player on headphones, get up and make a cup of tea, do some knitting - anything's better than lying there wishing you were asleep - and when you lie down again you may find you drop off immediately.

Nausea and vomiting
The exact cause of nausea and vomiting in pregnancy is not known but it is almost certainly linked to the hormonal changes taking place in the body and possibly due to psychological factors as well. Typically the expectant mother suffers from nausea and perhaps vomiting first thing in the morning from as early as six weeks to twelve or fourteen weeks, but this pattern varies greatly - in the degree of nausea felt, the time of day it comes on and how long it continues. It is rare for vomiting to become a serious problem and only in very few cases does it continue beyond about three months though it may recur in the last few weeks before the birth.

If you suffer from nausea eat little and often and avoid fried, fatty or spicy foods - or anything else that seems to set it off. Carbohydrates can help to alleviate it but don't use this as an excuse to tuck into too many buns: while some women understandably lose weight due to nauseousness, others put it on as they attempt to stave it off - not a good start to the well-managed pregnancy! On the other hand if you are actually vomiting a lot you will have to eat and more importantly drink when and what you can.

If early morning sickness is your problem keep some plain biscuits by the bedside and ask someone to make you a cup of tea to drink before you get out of bed, then wait for about ten minutes before getting up. Though usually recommended to mothers-to-be, milk can upset those who are nauseous. Drink plenty of other fluids, especially fruit juices in carbonated water: the sugar content and the bubbles should help you keep it down.

Don't worry about weight loss harming your baby - most women lose some weight in the first three months - but a loss of over about 4 or 5 kg should be reported to your doctor, as should severe vomiting - several times a day - or vomiting that persists after the fourteenth week or recurs later on. You may be prescribed an anti-emetic to relieve vomiting but not before about ten weeks because of the effects some such drugs have had in the past, for instance thalidomide.

Nosebleed

Because of your increased blood supply and progesterone nosebleeds are more frequent in pregnancy: the blood vessels in the mucous membrane of the nose dilate slightly and are more likely to rupture when you blow your nose. They are not a sign of high blood pressure (the old wives' story) and usually stop within a few minutes.

To stop bleeding bend your head slightly forward and pinch your nose gently. Wait for a full ten minutes, timed on a clock, before you stop pinching; if bleeding has not stopped, go on pinching for a little longer. Afterwards avoid blowing your nose if possible so as not to disturb the scab. Should you have a lot of trouble with nosebleeds the doctor may suggest that you have the blood vessels cauterized.

Pica

Interpreted as an abnormal and almost uncontrollable craving - stories of women eating soil and coal are most common - true pica is rare today but many women develop a strong liking for a particular food at some point during pregnancy. Provided this doesn't lead to an exclusive diet of one foodstuff, such cravings can do no harm.

It is thought that true pica is in fact brought on by a deficiency of iron or vitamins that the mother-to-be is trying to put right. If you find you do have a very strong desire for something odd mention this to the doctor at your

Skin changes
You can soothe itchy skin with calamine lotion, and by wearing clothes of cotton rather than man-made fabrics. Although there's no known cure for stretch marks, you can keep your skin in good condition by massaging it daily with cream containing lanolin or vitamin E. Oils containing vitamin E can be used instead - try adding a few drops of lavender oil to a neutral 'carrier' such as wheatgerm or almond oil, and using this for massage.

next ante-natal visit. In the unlikely event that it is due to some deficiency in your diet it can then be dealt with.

Skin changes

You may be lucky enough to enjoy the traditional glowing skin of the expectant mother. The response to hormonal changes in pregnancy, however, changes the skin in various ways. If you have a greasy skin it may become more greasy while those with dry skin find it even drier - the aggravated dryness is in fact very common and often associated with skin irritation which can get quite bad. Be extra scrupulous about keeping greasy skin clean and use plenty of moisturizer and bath oil to help prevent excessive dryness.

Some women get unaccustomed red spots and others a flushed look while pregnant. The skin also tends to tan more easily because it produces more pigment, and patches of darker skin (chloasma) may appear. Chloasma may come in the form of the so-called mask of pregnancy, shaped rather like a butterfly's wings over the face (this can be quite attractive or else blotchy and disfiguring). Moles, freckles, birthmarks and scars may all darken until after the birth and this effect will be increased by exposure to the sun, as will the chloasma. (Don't use a sunbed while you're pregnant as its possible effects on the fetus are not known.) A darkening of the skin round your nipples (the areola) and the appearance of a dark line (the linea nigra) running from the pubic area up to the navel (sometimes even higher) are further skin changes specific to pregnancy that usually fade again after the birth.

Unfortunately, although they do fade after the birth, the dreaded stretch marks do not disappear: what were reddish streaks on the breast and, more usually, belly only fade to a silvery white and cannot be got rid of. Neither can they reliably be prevented - oiling, massage and exercises to keep the skin supple only work up to a point. Stretch marks are caused by tearing in the less elastic lower layer of the skin. They can only be avoided by not overstretching this skin, that is, by not gaining too much weight but follow the advice of your doctor or midwife on this.

Sweating

Many women find they sweat more than usual, especially in the later stages of pregnancy, and find hot weather very hard to take. Once again, this is due to the dilatation of blood vessels caused by your increased blood supply and the problem will pass after the birth. In the meantime it's just a matter of trying to keep cool and calm and not over-exerting yourself unnecessarily. Take a cool shower and have a rest if you feel you're about to burst into a lather. Heavy sweating is particularly associated with bulk so keep an eye on your weight gain but drink plenty of fluids to make up for the extra lost by sweating.

Swelling

In itself swelling in pregnancy is neither unusual nor serious. The body retains fluid in varying amounts in different women - sometimes as much as six litres - and this puffs out the body tissue, collecting especially in the feet and legs. Mild swelling of the ankles at the end of the day, especially when it is hot, requires no treatment. If, however, swelling bothers you during the day, rest with your feet up and avoid prolonged standing. Wearing support tights can also help.

Greater facial fullness is common in pregnant women from the very start but increased puffiness can be a sign of too great a weight gain, fluid retention and is also a symptom of pre-eclampsia (a comon complaint in pregnancy which causes the blood pressure to rise, see page 90). Swelling and tightness in the wrist can cause Carpal Tunnel syndrome a disorder which gives rise to a numbing, tingling feeling in the fingers.

Report anything more than very mild swelling (when more severe it is known as oedema) at your ante-natal visit, especially if an impression is left after you have pressed the swollen area, particularly of the ankle, with your thumb. This is one of the signs of pre-eclampsia.

Oedema can be treated by controlling your diet to keep your weight down and also possibly a restriction on your intake of salt (which holds water).

Swelling
Take off any jewellery before it gets stuck, and rest during the day with your feet up if your ankles tend to swell. Naturopaths recommend eliminating salt from your diet, and taking regular exercise to help circulation. Dandelion is a natural way of dealing with fluid retention, but may not be terrifically effective - try using dandelion leaves in salad, or make a tea with them.

Massage to the affected areas can help, and a practitioner will use specific lymph drainage techniques. Acupuncture to the meridians of the kidneys and bladder is sometimes effective. As far as self-help is concerned, the key words are put your feet up.

When cystitis is responsible for frequent, painful urination, drink as much water as you can but avoid alcohol and strong coffee or tea. Make sure you wipe your anus from front to back, so that you don't transfer faecal bacteria to your urethra. Reducing your intake of animal protein and citrus fruits may help - so might avoiding acidic foods like tomatoes, rhubarb, gooseberries, vinegar and pickles.

Barleywater can be soothing - make it by boiling 100 g (4 oz) barley in a little water, then straining it. Pour 0.5 litre (1 pint) fresh water over the boiled barley, add the peel from half a lemon, and simmer gently until the barley is soft. Allow it to stand until it's cooled to blood heat, then remove the barley and add 50 g (2 oz) honey. Drink as much of it as you like.

Another useful herbal remedy is based on marshmallow root. Make a decoction by adding 25 g (1 oz) of the chopped or crushed root to 0.75 litre (1.5 pints) of distilled water, bring it to the boil in an enamel or stainless steel pan, and simmer until the liquid reduces to 0.5 litre (1 pint). Leave it to cool before straining it, and drink a cupful three times a day.

If pressures, chills or infections are responsible for

Urinary problems

A need to pass urine more frequently than usual is one of the earliest indications of pregnancy. Caused by the swelling uterus pressing on the bladder, it continues until the uterus rises up out of the pelvic cavity at about twelve weeks, giving the bladder more space again. It often recurs, however, in the last ten weeks, first when the baby's head is on the brim of the pelvis and then when it is engaged, both positions of which put pressure on the bladder.

At this time you may also suffer from incontinence - involuntary loss of urine - as the baby kicks out or as its head rotates against the pelvic brim, irritating the bladder. The prime cause of incontinence in pregnancy is weakness of the muscles in the pelvic floor. The hormone progesterone softens the ring of muscles that closes the bladder so that when you sneeze, cough or laugh or do anything to raise the pressure in the abdomen the ring relaxes and urine escapes (this is known as stress incontinence). The other main cause is infection of the urinary tract, made more likely by the action of progesterone which slackens the muscle walls of the bladder and the ureters between bladder and kidneys.

Needing to pass urine more often simply has to be put up with but you can do something about stress incontinence. There are exercises which strengthen the pelvic floor muscles and prevent stress incontinence during pregnancy which should be taken up again after the birth (which stretches the muscles, worsening the situation). Continue to do them for as long as you feel the need; unfortunately many mothers find stress incontinence becomes progressively worse with each succeeding pregnancy and birth if post-natal exercises are not done properly and regularly.

As for bladder infections - of which cystitis is the most common - if you experience pain before, during or after the urgent need to pass urine, see your doctor as soon as possible (there may also be a touch of blood in your urine). Cystitis should be treated promptly to ensure your good health; it won't directly affect the baby. You will probably be prescribed antibiotics. To help yourself, drink lots and lots of water until the infection has gone.

Vaginal discharge

About a third of expectant mothers will notice an increase in their vaginal secretions. There is cause for concern only if the discharge is heavy, coloured, smells unpleasant or there is soreness or irritation - it is probably caused by an infection. Otherwise it is purely a side-effect of changes in the mucous membrane of the vaginal tissues as they prepare for the dilatation of childbirth. Sometimes an increase in vaginal discharge at the end of pregnancy marks the onset of labour.

If you think you may have an infection tell your doctor. Thrush is the most common, caused by a fungus (*Candida albicans*) that thrives in a pregnant woman's extra-acid and sugary vagina. You will be treated with an anti-fungal ointment or pessary and can help yourself by eating unpasteurized yoghurt whose micro-organisms help to destroy the fungus and by adding a little bicarbonate of soda to your bath water to counter the acidity.

Reinfection is common and it is possible that both your partner and your baby (after its birth) will also require treatment. The baby catches it either as it passes through the vagina or from your skin when breastfeeding. It looks like tiny patches of curdled milk in the mouth and causes a nappy rash resistant to treatment. Don't worry about it but do get it seen to.

Varicose veins

Not only does the volume of blood increase in pregnancy and put extra strain on the veins but also the valve system, intended to prevent blood pooling in the lower limbs, often breaks down as the muscles of the vein wall relax under the influence of the hormone progesterone. Blood gathers in the legs, distending the veins there, and the situation is worsened by the enlarging uterus obstructing the flow of blood back from the legs to the heart.

A tendency to varicose veins is hereditary but stand-

inflammation of the bladder, acupuncture can identify the causes and treat them. Homoeopathic remedies vary, and are suited to individuals.

Vaginal discharge
If you're suffering from thrush, both you and your sexual partner should be treated as it's easily transmitted by intercourse. Wear cotton pants (wash them in non-biological washing powder) - and avoid tights, hot bubble baths and excessive washing with soaps and disinfectants. Adding bicarbonate of soda to your bathwater helps reduce acidity.

All 'alternative' therapies stress that attention to diet is the starting point for both prevention and treatment of thrush - it seems that diets high in sugars and refined carbohydrates are a primary cause. So cut down on sugars and starch, and avoid things like bread, cheese and alcohol which contain yeast. Eating plenty of foods containing vitamins A and E, and those of the B complex - plus zinc - is a good idea: if you're already enjoying a good wholefood diet you should be getting enough of these, but vegans may need vitamin and mineral supplements. Eat as much pasteurized yoghurt as you like. It contains micro-organisms that destroy the fungus and form a natural barrier against re-infection. According to naturopaths, garlic (either naturally or in tablet form) and olive oil attack the yeast-like fungus, and acidophilus (available in powder form, as tablets, or occurring naturally in some yoghurts) helps to restore your normal bacterial balance. Herbalists and homoeopaths treat thrush; remedies depend on individual needs so consult a practitioner.

Varicose veins

Self-help measures include putting on supporting tights before getting out of bed, not standing or sitting still for long periods and avoiding crossing your legs - even at the ankles. A good wholefood diet and daily exercise help to improve circulation, and prevent both excessive weight-gain and constipation. Herbalists suggest applying distilled witch hazel or tincture of calendula to the vein two or three times a day; hydrotherapy - contrast bathing with hot and cold water - will relieve any pain. Very gentle massage up the legs towards the heart, using 15 drops of essential oils of calendula or lavender to 50 ml (3 tablespoons) almond oil, is recommended by some practitioners - but consult an expert on this, as it may not be advisable in your case.

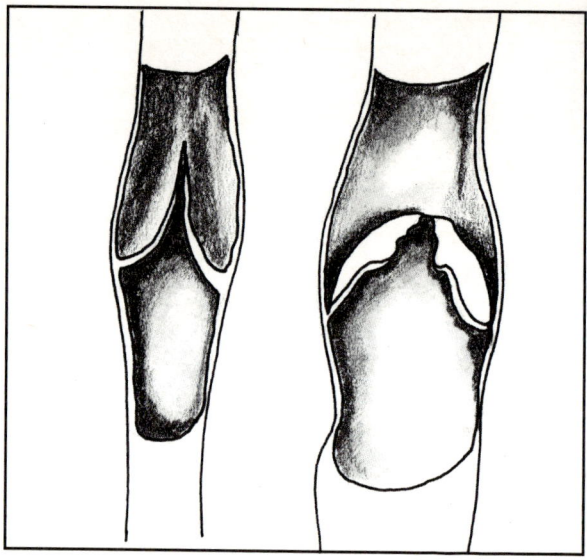

A normal vein has semi-lunar valves which allow blood to flow up, but prevent it flowing back. A vein becomes varicosed when the valve allows blood to seep back and pool within the vein.

ing still for long periods and carrying a lot of weight are major contributory factors (women bearing twins are particularly liable to them). If you have varicose veins they will get worse as the pregnancy advances but will improve afterwards, fading sometimes over a period of months. They do not always disappear completely, however, and will probably recur if you become pregnant again, getting progressively worse with each pregnancy.

Symptoms include slight irritation and itching, swelling of the feet and ankles and real discomfort in your legs as well as the unsightly veins themselves and, in severe cases, a shiny, smooth look to the skin.

Any action you can take is preventative only. To keep varicose veins at bay and/or prevent them from deteriorating, avoid standing still too often, gaining too much weight, and sitting with crossed legs (this further impedes the flow of blood in your legs). Take gentle exercise and if you have to stand shift your weight from foot to foot and contract your leg and foot muscles occasionally - do anything to encourage the blood to circulate. Sit with your feet and legs up whenever you can - even raise the foot of your bed a little (unless you've got heartburn as well!).

Wear elastic support tights until the veins have gone down after the birth and put these on as soon as you get up - not just when your legs begin to ache. Put them on straight after your bath or even before you stand up for the first time in the morning.

Common birth problems

Induction of labour

Where pregnancy has been prolonged for more than forty-two weeks the baby is called postmature and there may be concern for its wellbeing, usually because of what is known as placental insufficiency. The placenta reaches full maturity at 30 to 34 weeks then gradually deteriorates and may become inadequate to support the baby after full term (40 weeks), though it is generally agreed that it can do its job for up to 42 weeks. Doctors tend to be particularly concerned about this in older mothers, those over thirty or thirty-five, and will do regular tests to make sure that all is well in these last weeks. Checks on your estriol level are usual: the level of this hormone rises in pregnancy but drops immediately before labour begins, so a low level of estriol in your urine may be a sign that the placenta is no longer functioning fully and the baby is short of food and oxygen. The fetal heart will also be listened to at regular intervals to check that this is satisfactory.

On the strength of such tests the doctor may decide to induce labour at some certain date if you have not already gone into labour naturally by then. Should you be unhappy about this decision, take comfort from the fact that many women enter hospital for an induction only to start off spontaneously once they're in! Where it is decided to induce labour you will be admitted to hospital the previous day.

It is not fully known why labour starts naturally, but to trigger it off artificially various methods are used (methods which may also be used to speed up a slow labour where contractions are weak).

Prostaglandin

A gel, cream or, more often, a pessary containing synthetic prostaglandin - similar to hormones found naturally in the uterus lining - is introduced into the vagina. This may be enough to stimulate labour but sometimes more than one dose is necessary and these pessaries are sometimes used at intervals over two to three days. Prostaglandin pessaries are also used just to soften the cervix for later induction by other means.

This is a fairly sympathetic method of induction: it is not too intrusive and leaves you free to move about.

Oxytocin

This is a natural hormone from the pituitary gland in the brain which is now produced synthetically (Syntocinon). It may be used to induce or speed up labour as well as in conjunction with the artificial breaking of the membranes or following on a dose of prostaglandin.

Oxytocin is usually given as an injection, a tablet or by intravenous drip (most common). If you are prescribed a tablet put it under your tongue or between cheek and gum and let it dissolve very slowly. If a drip is to be inserted ask for a long tube so you can move around more easily, though of course you will be restricted to the bed. The drip stays in place throughout labour to make sure the contractions continue - as they would naturally - to deliver the placenta as well as the baby and to prevent bleeding.

Oxytocin has the advantage of acting almost immediately but strong contractions can come on so fast and with so little space between them it is quite a shock to the mother who has had no gradual build-up to get used to the pain and this may lead to a greater resort to pain-killing drugs.

Artificial Rupture of the Membrane (ARM)

Again often used together with other means of induction, amniotomy (ARM) is the artificial breaking of the membranes (releasing the waters) by use of forceps or a special crochet-hook type instrument. This is inserted into the uterus and the process is no more than uncomfortable, indeed completely painless if the cervix is slightly dilated already.

Amniotomy brings on labour quickly and the nearer the mother is to term the sooner it starts. It may work because the pressure inside the uterus has altered or because the now 'uncushioned' head of the baby presses on the cervix and encourages the uterus to contract. But the membranes are not usually ruptured unless you are near your due date, mainly because of the risk of infection which means the baby must be delivered within twenty-four hours.

Amniotomy may also be done when labour is already underway, to speed it up, and sometimes because the medical staff want to monitor the baby via an electrode on his head.

Controversy

Opinions vary enormously over induction of labour. Many people feel that the baby should decide when it arrives and that there is far too much interference in childbirth. Where labour is artificially induced your chances of further intervention - in the form perhaps of a forceps delivery or a Cesarean - are certainly increased. On the other hand, where there is some chance, however small, that the baby is at risk it is hard to argue against delivery as soon as possible. Birth is often induced in high-risk pregnancies, for instance where the mother carries twins or has diabetes or high blood pressure. What most mothers object to is being induced for the convenience of doctors and medical staff - very few would choose to be induced for their own convenience - although where medical intervention is going to be necessary, for example where there is a Rhesus incompatibility, this does make sense.

Assisted delivery

A long and difficult labour brings danger of fetal or maternal distress and delivery is often hastened by various means. The second stage in particular is not usually allowed to continue for more than an hour and a half after which time the doctor will intervene with forceps or vacuum extractor or, if appropriate, by performing a Cesarean section.

Forceps

Invented about 400 years ago, forceps provided the first mechanical aid used in childbirth. Those used today have separate stainless steel blades that fit neatly round each side of the baby's head making a sort of protective cage around it. The two blades are actually inserted one side at a time then the handles are joined together in such a way that they lock the blades firmly. When the forceps are in place the doctor uses them either to rotate the baby's head (if it is in the wrong position) or to pull gently on it to assist delivery; he does this during contractions only.

Vacuum extractor

Also known as a ventouse, this does more or less the same job as forceps. A small metal cup connected to a vacuum pump is placed on the baby's head and a vacuum then created inside the cup which makes it stick firmly to the head. The doctor can then use a handle on the tubing connected to the cup to turn or to pull on the baby.

There is little to choose between forceps and vacuum extraction but the latter does have the advantage of involving less intrusion into the vagina with, consequently, less risk of damaging the mother or of introducing infection. On the other hand the forceps serve to protect the head as it is delivered and they are sometimes used on premature babies and always in breech deliveries for this reason.

If the ventouse is used, there is usually less need for an episiotomy because it doesn't take up extra space round the baby's head like the forceps. Forceps can only be applied where the cervix is fully dilated. Both methods leave the baby marked - with forceps red marks on cheeks and ears, with the ventouse a red swollen area on the crown of the head where the vacuum cup fitted - but in both cases the marks disappear in a few days.

Delivery is assisted by using one of the above when labour is taking a long time because the baby's head is difficult to deliver. The head may be large in relation to the mother's pelvis or the baby may be facing his mother's navel rather than her spine - the usual and straightforward position - in which case the doctor may attempt to turn the baby round. (When the baby is in this position, called occipito posterior, contractions often slow down so it may be necessary to help the baby out.)

An assisted delivery is required for a breech birth

(buttocks first) especially where the mother has an epidural. In fact epidurals in general often mean some help will be needed because they tend to reduce the mother's urge and ability to push as well as slowing down contractions. Finally, forceps or ventouse are introduced where the mother is too tired to push any longer or where the doctor feels she should not be bearing down because of risk to her own health, for instance if she has high blood pressure or heart disease.

Assisted delivery requires an anesthetic, usually local, sometimes general. Afterwards the mother often is bruised and sore, especially with forceps, and she may also feel violated and angry with medical staff as well as disappointed with herself for requiring intervention. Some feel nothing but relief that labour is over and a healthy baby delivered.

Cesarean section

From the Latin caedere, to cut, a Cesarean involves cutting through the abdominal wall and through the lower part of the uterus, removing the baby and afterbirth and stitching up the incisions. It takes just five minutes from the first cut to the birth of the baby. The Cesarean has not always been the safe operation it is today and it saves babies, and mothers, who might otherwise have been damaged or even died. It is widely felt, however, that it is too readily resorted to where there is a problem, and it should not be forgotten that it is still a major operation with all the attendant risks.

A Cesarean may be either elective - arranged in advance because of known complications - or an emergency - undertaken once labour is under way, when a problem arises. The former may be done either under general anesthetic or with an epidural but with an emergency there is not enough time to set up an epidural so the operation will be done under general anesthetic unless of course you have already opted for an epidural for your labour.

An elective Cesarean section is always performed in cases of placenta praevia (where the placenta is obstructing the cervical opening); where the baby's head is too big to fit through the mother's pelvis; if it is a breech birth (when there is a risk that the baby's head, delivered after the body, will press against the umbilical cord in the pelvic opening, cutting off its own oxygen supply). Pre-eclampsia (rare) and actual eclampsia (very rare) are also indications for Cesarean section as is transverse lie, where the baby is lying at right angles to the mother's spine and it has not been possible to turn him. A Cesarean will sometimes be performed instead of the use of forceps; indeed, it has largely replaced the more difficult types of forceps deliveries.

Afterwards you have an operation to recover from, with the effects of the anesthetic and pain in the scar plus minor discomforts such as wind. You may be on an intravenous drip for 24 hours but will be encouraged to move about as soon as possible. Stitches or clips come out after about a week and you will probably be home within ten days. It can take anything from six weeks to six months for complete recovery - this is usually sooner rather than later where the Cesarean was performed under an epidural.

Episiotomy

This is a cut made during labour between the vaginal opening and the anus (perineum) to prevent tearing and to help get the baby out quickly where the vaginal outlet is too tight. There is no doubt that there are occasions when an episiotomy is called for, for instance where forceps are to be used, but opinions differ as to whether episiotomy is essential in most labours.

The cut is made with scissors during a contraction as the baby's head stretches the tissues of the perineum and is stitched up once the placenta has been delivered, usually with dissolvable stitches. Both incision and stitching (called suturing in hospitals) are done under local anesthetic and are not too painful.

After the birth

Once over the hurdle of the birth most of us assume that

now all will go smoothly but unfortunately it does not always, especially with a first baby. Furthermore, when you do come up against a problem, it is all too easy to let it throw you completely rather than keeping it in perspective and coping.

Breastfeeding

Worry, together with lack of experience, is often at the root of problems that arise with breastfeeding and that, sadly, can lead to mothers giving it up. Anxiety about breastfeeding, primarily whether your baby is getting enough milk, can in itself reduce your milk supply. Problems at the outset, like the general discomfort you still feel after the birth and weariness caused by the little rest and privacy available in hospital combine with your lack of confidence - which the nurses are not always sympathetic to - such that your brain may not send the right messages to the breasts and the 'let-down' reflex (which triggers the release of milk) doesn't occur. If this happens, your baby doesn't get the more nutritious hindmilk, cries because he or she is hungry causing you to worry more, setting up a vicious circle.

Try to relax - and make sure your baby gets to feed for long enough (it can take a couple of minutes in some women for the let-down reflex to work) and lastly ensure that he takes the whole nipple right inside his mouth to feed as this is also necessary to stimulate the reflex.

Engorgement

When the milk 'comes in' on the third or fourth day you may find that overnight you have bursting breasts, tender and sometimes painful. To relieve the engorgement the most important thing is to continue feeding your baby; if he finds it difficult to latch on to your swollen breasts express a little milk by hand just before feeding - stroking the breasts under a warm shower or putting hot flannels on them makes the milk flow more easily.

Cracked nipples

Really sore nipples sometimes develop a painful crack.

Avoid feeding from this breast and express milk instead until it heals. Keep the nipple dry and expose the breast to the air as much as possible.

Mastitis

If the crack or blocked duct becomes infected the area will be red and tender, you will have a temperature and may feel rather fluish.

Rest, in bed if you can, but continue feeding the baby, giving the sore breast first to make sure all the milk is cleared from it. Express the milk if you cannot feed. You may need antibiotics. Don't ignore the problem as it can lead to a nasty abscess within the breast which may require surgery to drain it although sometimes a course of antibiotic alone is enough.

Post-natal depression

It is almost inevitable that a new mother will feel rather weepy about three or four days after the birth, almost as a reaction to the build-up in tension of the pregnancy and the powerful experience of the birth. Most new mothers have some anxieties and difficulties: perhaps they feel they'll never be able to cope with their demanding baby and re-establish relations with their partner and then there are worries about loneliness, money, loss of independence - everything assumes greater importance than it deserves in the eyes of someone who is not getting enough sleep!

However, sometimes this normal muddle of understandable concerns, rather than dissipating as you regain control, develops into serious depression with overwhelming lethargy and inability to cope. If you find you are continually weepy, feel completely exhausted, inadequate and irritable, perhaps even uninterested in your baby, and talking to your partner or to friends doesn't help, seek professional advice. See your doctor or a psychotherapist; there may also be a post-natal support group near you that you could contact. Do something, don't just sit at home and despair: ask for help.

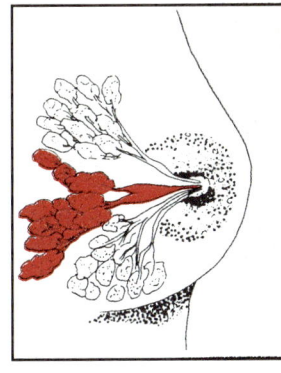

Blocked ducts
Sometimes a lump forms in the breast where a milk duct has become blocked. To clear it, feed more frequently, stroke the breast towards the nipple under a warm shower or after applying oil, and feed your baby in a different position so he draws on all parts of the breast.

Serious complications

Miscarriage

Once the final pre-pregnancy menstrual period is past expectant mothers dread vaginal bleeding as an almost invariable sign of trouble - and indeed they are quite right to do so, at whatever stage of pregnancy, and especially when it is accompanied by abdominal pain. Bleeding may sometimes threaten trouble that doesn't materialize or, taken as a warning, may lead to effective preventative action, such as bed rest, but unfortunately it can also mean that you lose your baby. Before the 28th week the loss of a baby is called a miscarriage or spontaneous abortion; after this it is known as a stillbirth.

Even a late period may be a very early miscarriage, where a fertilized egg has failed to implant in the uterus. In the first ten weeks of pregnancy miscarriage is likely to be due to abnormal development of the embryo. However, many women give birth to fine, healthy babies after blood spotting and even after more than one instance of real, quite severe, loss of blood. When a threatened miscarriage continues as a normal pregnancy there is absolutely no reason to fear any abnormality.

The first sign of a threatened miscarriage is bleeding, which may get worse gradually or may be heavy from the start and accompanied by cramps like period pains. Cramping pains, caused by the uterus contracting, are more of a danger sign than just bleeding but a degree of dull aching pain should not be worried about. Similarly, the loss of clots of blood is serious where a flow of blood is not so much so.

Phone your doctor at once if you are concerned. You will probably be advised to take to your bed for a few days and this is enough in the great majority of cases to stem the flow. In the remainder, both bleeding and cramps increase (even if you are resting) until the fetus is expelled. After this you will probably need to go to hospital for an operation to make sure that everything is cleared out from the uterus (D & C: dilation and curettage) unless the bleeding stops very quickly as it does sometimes in an early miscarriage.

Hormone deficiency

If you have previously miscarried you may be tested for a deficiency of progesterone (which should be produced in adequate amounts by the corpus luteum then by the placenta) and put on a course if this should it prove necessary.

Missed abortion

Here the embryo dies very early on but the uterus fails to expel it and the placenta continues to grow, leading to a positive pregnancy test result. The 'pregnancy' may continue for as long as fourteen weeks but eventual miscarriage is inevitable.

Habitual miscarriage

Most miscarriages are not followed up but where someone miscarries three or more times at more or less the same stage, investigations will be made to determine the cause. It may or may not be possible to settle on a cause - or to do anything about it - but there is one instance at least where preventative action can be taken in a subsequent pregnancy - where there is cervical incompetence.

Incompetent cervix

On rare occasions bleeding in mid-pregnancy (after 12 weeks and often at about 20 weeks) is due to cervical incompetence where the muscle round the neck of the uterus is weak - either naturally or as a result of damage during a previous birth or vaginal operation, particularly termination - and isn't doing its proper job of holding the fetus within the uterus. Bleeding is often accompanied by loss of the amniotic fluid as the membranes bulge out of the cervix then break. A miscarriage or premature birth, though usually painless, is inevitable depending on when this happens; there is no cure.

There is however an efficient preventative measure though this will have to wait for your next pregnancy. After an internal examination or ultrasound scan has confirmed the diagnosis of incompetent cervix a special stitch is put in it. This is done under general anesthetic at about 12 to 14 weeks and will keep the cervix closed until

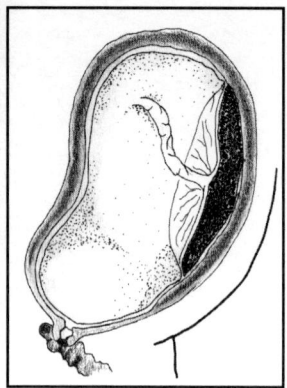

Normal placenta position

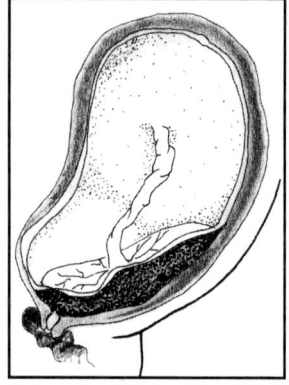

Placenta praevia

it is removed at about 36-38 weeks. Cutting this stitch, known as a Shirodkar suture (named after the Indian doctor who first performed it), does not require anesthetic and gives no more than slight discomfort. After this labour may start either at once or not until full term. Should labour begin before the stitch is removed this can be done immediately and easily.

Placenta praevia/abruptio

Bleeding in the second half of pregnancy may be due either to the placenta being unsuitably positioned in the uterus near or sometimes over the cervix (placenta praevia) or to it becoming detached from the uterus wall (placenta abruptio).

In the first case the placenta, because it is implanted in the lower part of the uterus, is inevitably separated at least partially from the uterus wall as this softens and eventually opens in preparation for labour. In the second, a normally positioned placenta separates prematurely from the uterus. If either is suspected an ultrasound scan may be used to decide between the two (placenta praevia is usually painless but placenta abruptio causes pain).

Neither condition is common, the latter even less than the former, but if you have bleeding, especially after 28 weeks, it is vital that you report it at once. A woman with placenta praevia will be kept in hospital to rest and any further bleeding investigated and dealt with in whatever way considered best for mother and child, for example, early delivery. In most cases a Cesarean section is necessary at the birth.

Treatment for placenta abruptio is rest in hospital with painkillers and monitoring of the fetal heart with an emergency Cesarean if the separation becomes so great that it is thought that the baby is not receiving enough food and oxygen.

Stillbirth

Spontaneous miscarriages even as early as 12 weeks can be distressing to the parents who were so full of pleasurable anticipation. Not only for the mother whose whole body and mind have undergone such great changes in preparation, but for the father too who is not usually as well-informed as to what may go wrong. Even where a baby was not planned, death in the uterus is a shock and its loss mourned. But to have a baby die in the later stages can be infinitely more traumatic.

The signs that a baby has died in the uterus are straightforward: lack of movement and, when checked, the lack of heart beat - though babies do often stop moving for no apparent reason for periods up to 24 hours. Further indications are negative: the mother losing weight, her breasts getting smaller again and any swelling on the body disappearing: the uterus shrinks.

When the diagnosis is confirmed labour may be induced - though it may begin spontaneously and sometimes the mother prefers to wait even some time for this to happen. It is up to the not-now-expectant mother to decide, with counselling, and she should receive the greatest consideration in all decisions at this time.

After the initial shock and numbness - and there is all the usual post-labour discomfort to cope with as well - the mother's reaction is typically one of both guilt and anger as well as of acute deprivation. Readjusting to not being pregnant, seeing other people's new babies and wondering if you could ever face the risk of going through it again are among other problems to be overcome. Coming to terms with a baby's death can take a very long time, though of course everyone reacts differently and the feeling of emptiness may be harder to bear where, for instance, you have no other children to keep you busy and on whom to lavish your tenderness.

Some women become seriously depressed after a stillbirth - and indeed after a miscarriage - and may need professional advice and attention should the support of her family and friends not prove enough. Many of the reactions described above will also apply where an induced abortion, or termination, has been sought, for whatever reason, though women who have had terminations for medical reasons are likely to suffer even longer-lasting and severe problems.

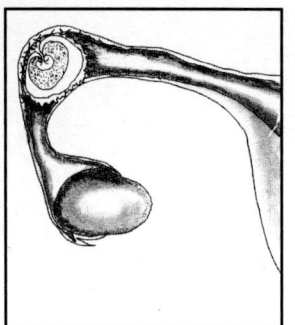

An ectopic pregnancy occurs when, instead of implanting and growing in the endometrium, the fertilized ovum implants in the fallopian tube itself. It grows until it eventually ruptures the tube which causes acute abdominal pain and internal bleeding.

Ectopic pregnancy

Any expectant mother who develops severe abdominal pain, perhaps on one side only, with slight bleeding, in the early days of her pregnancy should report this at once to her doctor in case she has an ectopic pregnancy. This means that instead of travelling down into the uterus the fertilized egg has implanted in one of the fallopian tubes.

The symptoms of pregnancy are normal as the usual hormones are produced and the embryo begins to develop. However, the tube cannot stretch as the uterus can so as the embryo grows it eats into the tube wall which will eventually rupture, causing bleeding and presenting a serious threat to the mother's health, life even. This would usually happen between the sixth and twelfth week. Urgent admission to hospital is necessary so that the affected tube may be removed under general anaesthetic together with its mistaken growth. This means that you cannot conceive on this side again though the fallopian tube can occasionally be repaired instead, once the embryo is removed.

If you have once had an ectopic pregnancy you should report for ante-natal examination as soon as you become pregnant again; an internal examination can usually tell if the egg has situated itself correctly or not, and ultrasound scanning may also be employed to look for the embryonic growth where an ectopic implantation is suspected.

Other problems may also loom during your pregnancy but are more readily spotted and held in check thanks to the high standards of modern ante-natal care.

Pre-eclampsia and high blood pressure

The importance of pre-eclampsia (which cannot be too greatly emphasized) is that it precedes eclampsia, a dangerous illness specific to pregnancy where convulsions can lead to death for both mother and baby because of a reduced supply of oxygen.

The exact cause of pre-eclampsia is not known although its signs and symptoms and some predisposing factors are. They include high blood pressure, swelling (edema) of the body, especially of hands and ankles, caused by fluid retention, and the presence of protein in the urine, and throughout pregnancy you will be checked for these at every ante-natal visit so don't forget to take a specimen every time you see the doctor or midwife. Your weight is also always noted as excessive weight gain has a bearing on the condition, especially after the twentieth week when pre-eclampsia is likely to occur.

Pre-eclampsia develops slowly and gradually and because of the close check kept for signs and symptoms can almost always be avoided. But if it is allowed to develop, that is, if symptoms are not dealt with by rest, altering the diet and possibly by drugs to bring down blood pressure, then headaches, blurring of vision and flashing lights before the eyes follow. These are real danger signs.

In itself pre-eclampsia is not harmful in the long term to the mother - after the birth the symptoms simply disappear - but it must be controlled lest it develop further into actual eclampsia. It can however be harmful to the baby: the higher the mother's blood pressure the more risk there is to the baby because of the likelihood of placental insufficiency. This would mean labour being induced or the baby being delivered by Cesarean section - even as early as 28 to 30 weeks - bringing all the risks and problems attached to babies born before term.

Rhesus incompatibility

Another problem of pregnancy that can almost always be dealt with satisfactorily today, provided the mother seeks ante-natal care, is that of Rhesus incompatibility.

The great majority of the population (85%) is Rhesus positive, which means that its red blood cells carry the Rhesus factor (Rh+). The remainder is Rhesus negative (Rh-). No problem arises until a Rh- woman has a baby with a Rh+ man in which case, again, there is no problem unless the baby (which inherits half of its genes from its father) is also Rh+. If this happens some of the baby's red blood cells pass into the mother's bloodstream during pregnancy and delivery, provoking the mother's blood to produce antibodies to destroy the 'foreign' Rh+ blood cells. (This may also happen if a woman has a miscarried or terminated baby or even an amniocentesis or Rh+ blood transfusion. In each of these cases blood from the fetus can mix with that of the mother.)

This action does not harm that first baby but in a subsequent pregnancy these antibodies will cross the placenta and, should the next baby be Rh+ as well, attack its red blood cells until the baby becomes so anemic that it dies either before or soon after birth. These deaths were a mystery until the 1940s when the Rhesus factor was discovered and a connection made with them. Today women are tested at their first ante-natal visit to see if they are RH- or RH+. If they are Rh- then the baby's blood will be tested; if this proves to be Rh+ the mother will be injected with antibodies (known as anti-D immunoglobin) within 12 hours of the birth (or miscarriage, termination or amniocentesis). These antibodies will attack any of the baby's Rh+ cells that have got into the mother's blood and destroy them before the mother's blood can develop its own antibodies. The problem is permanently solved as in subsequent pregnancy she has no antibodies to harm her Rh+ baby should she have one.

Should a mother slip through the net of ante-natal care, or have developed antibodies before pregnancy (unlikely but possible) the baby's heart will be regularly monitored by ultrasound scanning and the degree of anemia by amniocentesis. Birth may be induced early or, should the baby be at great risk, it may be given a blood transfusion even before it is born. After the birth, less severely affected babies will be treated by phototherapy or be given a complete exchange of blood.

Prematurity

A baby is usually considered to be premature if born before the thirty-sixth week of pregnancy. The fetus is considered viable in law at 28 weeks but babies now survive when born as early as 24 weeks where they are lucky enough to have expert nursing in an intensive care unit.

It is not always known why a particular baby has

arrived prematurely but it may be because of abnormality of the placenta, incompetent cervix, ill-health or poor diet or anemia in the mother, ovarian cysts and fibroids or abnormalities of the uterus. Twins - and multiples - are also more likely to be premature. Also in some cases of diabetes, high blood pressure and pre-eclampsia, labour may be induced early because however hard the baby may have to struggle for life outside the uterus he has more of a chance than he has inside. This is in spite of the fact that normally every week, even day, the baby remains in the uterus his chances of surviving improve, mainly because the lungs are not properly developed pre-term. In cases where premature labour before 32 weeks seems inevitable, drugs may be given to the mother to delay it a day or so to allow time to give the baby cortisone injections to stimulate his lung development and reduce the risk of breathing problems after the birth.

Labour

As a premature baby's skull is softer than that of a full-term baby labour is often both shorter and easier. The baby's head, however, may need to be protected from damage by using forceps or doing an episiotomy more readily so that the natural gripping and squeezing of the cervix and vagina are applied to the forceps rather than directly to the baby's skull. An epidural is used for pain relief where possible as drugs such as pethidine or a general anesthetic (for a Cesarean section) may upset the baby.

Treatment

The premature baby's main problems are those of:
• Breathing - he may develop respiratory distress which is dealt with by giving him oxygen or in severe cases 'ventilating' him artificially by means of a tube in his windpipe;
• Temperature control - babies are usually placed in thermostatically controlled incubators to keep their body temperature steady;
• Infection - the incubator and cleanliness of the unit

Signs of fetal distress
• The passing of green meconium from the baby's bowels, normally passed after birth (though this does occasionally happen in a straightforward labour).
• Changes in the fetal heart rate: it should beat fairly steadily, though slowing during a contraction, at about 140 beats a minute. An irregular and very high or very low beat is suspect.
• Sudden and fierce movements of the baby during labour. Where fetal distress is feared a blood sample may be taken from the baby's scalp and tested to see its oxygen level. The heart will be monitored.

largely isolates him from infection but his resistance can best be built up by breast milk, though this may have to be given via a tube if he is too weak to suck.

One thing is certain, the survival rate for premature babies has increased dramatically in the last ten years, and only a tiny minority of those that survive suffer any sort of physical or mental handicap.

Hemorrhage

Blood loss of up to 500 ml (approximately one pint) is considered normal during and after delivery of the placenta in the third stage of labour but excessive bleeding is usually stopped by the contractions of the uterus constricting the blood vessels. Sometimes the uterus cannot contract to do this job because the placenta has not completely come away from the uterus wall.

Giving the mother oxytocin by injection to encourage the uterus to contract (and putting the baby to the breast so that natural oxytocin may be released) is usually enough to expel the fragment and stop the bleeding but sometimes it may have to be removed under epidural or general anesthetic if bleeding is severe.

Where a woman suffers hemorrhaging after the birth - perhaps up to five or ten days later - it is usually for the same reason and dealt with similarly or it may be due to an infection in the uterus in which case antibiotics are prescribed.

Bleeding may also result from tearing of the cervix or vagina which will need stitching or, very rarely, because of a deficiency in the mother's blood clotting mechanism - for instance after placenta abruptio where all the clotting factors in her blood may have been 'used up' trying to control the bleeding from the placenta.

Fetal distress

This term means that the baby is short of oxygen and during labour this shortage may become acute, for instance if the umbilical cord has twisted round the baby's neck or become knotted, restricting or cutting off the blood supply, or if the placenta has sheared off from the uterine wall (placenta abruptio).

The baby may also run short of oxygen because the contractions are coming fast, one close after the other. Every contraction obstructs the supply of blood to the placenta as the blood vessels in the uterus wall are constricted. Normally the baby draws on the reserve of blood in the placenta to cope with this. A healthy baby also has the ability to survive for up to ten minutes without oxygen. After a time, however, any baby will suffer without oxygen and this may eventually result in brain damage or even death. Where a baby is small and/or malnourished for any reason, or perhaps the placenta is not working efficiently, it may be that he has no reserves to draw on and will become distressed sooner.

If fetal distress is severe and labour progressing slowly, a Cesarean section will usually be performed; in less urgent cases or where labour is at a later stage an episiotomy, forceps or ventouse may be used to speed up delivery and get the baby safely out. Afterwards the baby will be observed to make sure he has suffered no ill-effects and may need extra care and attention.

Other titles in the series

Your Active Body (ISBN 0 245-55070-4)
Your Sex Life (ISBN 0 245-55067-4)
Your Heart and Lungs (ISBN 0 245-55069-0)

Available, Spring 1990
Your Mind (ISBN 0 245-60008-6)
Your Diet (ISBN 0 245-60009-4)
Your Skin (ISBN 0 245-60010-8)
Your Child (ISBN 0 245-60011-6)

Available, Autumn 1990
Your Female Body (ISBN 0 245-60012-4)
Your Senses (ISBN 0 245-60013-2)
A-Z of Conditions and Drugs (ISBN 0 245-60014-0)

Useful organizations

*Family Planning Information
Service
27-35 Mortimer Street
London W1N 7RJ*

*National Childbirth Trust
9 Queensborough Terrace
London W2 3TB*

*Natural Family Planning
Centre
Queen Elizabeth Medical
Centre
Edgbaston
Birmingham B15 2TG*

*Pregnancy Advisory Service
11-13 Charlotte Street
London W1P 1ND*

*Gingerbread
2nd Floor
35 Wellington Street
London WC2E 7BN*

*Women's Health Information
Centre
52-54 Featherstone Street
London EC1Y 8RT*

*Stillbirth and Neonatal Deaths
Society
28 Portland Place
London W1N 3DE*

*Society of Homoeopaths
47 Canada Grove
Bognor Regis
West Sussex PO21 1OW*

*Council for Acupuncture
(umbrella group for the main
colleges)
Suite One
191A Cavendish Squre
London W1M 9AD*

*General Council and Register
of Osteopaths
21 Suffolk Street
London SW1Y 4HG*

*National Institute of Medical
Herbalists
41 Hatherley Road
Winchester
Hampshire SO22 6RR*

*PRIME HEALTH
Private Medical Insurers
Prime House
Barnett Wood Lane
Leatherhead
Surrey KT22 7BS
0372 386060*